THE FAM
HOME REM
COLLECT

D0355106

Curing
Common
Complaints

THE FAMILY
HOME REMEDIES
COLLECTION

CURING
COMMON
COMPLAINTS

From bad breath to fatigue,
heartburn and tooth stains, the
best doctor-tested tips to
relieve everyday health concerns

BY THE EDITORS OF
PREVENTION MAGAZINE HEALTH BOOKS

Rodale Press, Emmaus, Pennsylvania

Book Packager: Sandra J. Taylor
Cover and Book Designer: Eugenie Seidenberg Delaney

Library of Congress Cataloging-in-Publication Data

Curing common complaints : from bad breath to fatigue, heartburn and tooth stains, the best doctor-tested tips to relieve everyday health concerns / by the editors of Prevention Magazine Health Books.
      p.   cm. — (The Family home remedies collection)
    Includes index.
    ISBN 0–87596–262–9 paperback
    1. Medicine, Popular. I. Prevention Magazine Health Books.
II. Series.
RC81.C925   1995
610—dc20   94–24201
                                          CIP

Distributed in the book trade by St. Martin's Press

2 4 6 8 10 9 7 5 3 1   paperback

———— OUR MISSION ————

We publish books that empower people's lives.

———— RODALE 🌱 BOOKS ————

NOTICE

This book is intended as a reference volume only, not as a medical guide or manual for self-treatment. If you suspect that you have a medical problem, please seek competent medical care. The information here is designed to help you make informed choices about your health. It is not intended as a substitute for any treatment prescribed by your doctor.

CONTENTS

ATHLETE'S FOOT

C onsidering that this ailment is most often associated with stalwart Schwarzeneggerites, it's no wonder that most people *don't* refer to athlete's foot by its wimpy clinical name: "ringworm of the feet."

But truth be told, this nasty little bugger could care less whether you pump up or punk out, whether your running is done in marathons or just into the kitchen for a halftime snack. If you want to see what encourages ringworm of the feet, just look down. Whether Nikes or ortho-walkers are your preferred footwear, they're ringworm's idea of a happy home.

"Athlete's foot is caused by a fungus that thrives in warm, moist conditions—and the closed shoes present a good 'incubator' for these organisms," says Michael Ramsey, M.D., clinical instructor of dermatology at Baylor College of Medicine in Houston. "That's why athlete's foot is quite uncommon in primitive cultures where shoes are not worn." But if you wear shoes more often than a bushman does, here's how to get a toehold on this irritating but relatively harmless infection.

Sock it to 'em. "Whenever you take off or put on your socks, it's a good practice to rub a sock up and down your toe webs," says Rodney Basler, M.D., assistant professor of internal medicine at the University of Nebraska Medical Center in Omaha. "That keeps the areas between your toes dry, which is essential in preventing and treating athlete's foot."

Get cooking with baking soda. Baking soda is a cheaper alternative to expensive foot powders, yet it does essentially the same thing. Either sprinkle it on dry or make a paste by moistening one tablespoon of baking soda with lukewarm water, suggests Suzanne M. Levine, D.P.M., a clinical assistant podiatrist at the Wycoff Heights Medical Center and adjunct clinical instructor at New York College of Podiatric Medicine, both in New York City. Rub the mixture on your feet and between your toes. After about 15 minutes, rinse it off and dry thoroughly.

The answer is blowin' from your dryer. "Use your hair dryer on your feet to dry them more effectively than you can with a towel," adds Dr. Basler. "And blowing air from your hair dryer into your shoes is a good way to dry them out after you wear them."

Find relief in sheep's clothing. "Placing lamb's wool between the tips of your toes [after removing your shoes] allows air to reach the affected skin, which helps make conditions less favorable for fungal growth," says Dr. Ramsey. So if the day's almost over and you can kick back for a while, prop up your bare feet with some lamb's wool between your toes.

Vote "pro" for antiperspirants. "Rubbing or spraying antiperspirant on your feet can keep them from sweating," says Dr. Basler. "You can use the same brand you use on your underarms. As long as it contains aluminum chlorohydrate, the active drying ingredient, it will work."

Disinfect your shoes. Neal Kramer, D.P.M., a Bethlehem, Pennsylvania, podiatrist, says that Lysol and other household disinfectants can kill off any living fungus spores. After you take off your shoes, rub the insides with a cloth or paper towel that has a dab of disinfectant. (Then use that hair dryer to dry out the insides of the shoes!)

The right solution: Don't use creams. Antifungal creams have the right ingredients but the wrong way of presenting them. "The problem with creams is that they *help* trap moisture, especially between toes," says Dr. Basler. "Solutions are much better than creams."

Use the power in powder. If you're going with an over-the-counter powder—the most common remedy—Dr. Ramsey says some of the best are Zeasorb-AF, Desenex, Tinactin and Micatin. "I recommend *against* using cornstarch, because it sometimes sets you up for a yeast infection," adds Dr. Basler, who also recommends Mycelex as a nonprescription remedy.

IS IT REALLY ATHLETE'S FOOT?

Y ou may be able to run like the wind, pump iron until it rusts and make your heart beat faster than Dan Cupid's target practice, but even the most versatile jock-of-all-trades is a lousy Marcus Welby when it comes to diagnosing athlete's foot.

"A lot of people who think they have athlete's foot actually have another condition—usually eczema, dermatitis or some kind of allergic reaction to their shoes," says Rodney Basler, M.D., assistant professor of internal medicine at the University of Nebraska Medical Center in Omaha. "One way to tell if it's *really* athlete's foot is if there's an infection in the toe web between your fourth and fifth toe—your 'ring' toe and pinkie. If it's *not* there, the problem is usually *not* athlete's foot."

It's also not athlete's foot if:

- The infection is identical on both feet. "Then it's probably eczema or an allergic reaction to your shoes," says Dr. Basler.
- It's only on the top of your toes. "Contact dermatitis may be caused by shoe material," he adds.
- It occurs on a child below the age of puberty. Athlete's foot rarely strikes before adolescence.
- The foot is red, swollen, blistered and sore. Again, severe dermatitis is the likely culprit.

Foot brine is fine. A mixture of two teaspoons of salt per pint of warm water provides a foot soak that zaps excess perspiration and hampers fungus growth, says Glenn Copeland, D.P.M., who is podiatrist for the Toronto Blue Jays professional baseball team and a staff member at the Toronto Women's College Hospital. Simply soak your feet for five to ten minutes at a time, repeating often until the condition clears. *Added bonus:* This saline solution helps soften the affected area, so antifungal medications can penetrate deeper for better results.

Remove dead skin. When your condition starts to improve, remove any dead skin. According to Frederick Hass, M.D., a general practitioner in San Rafael, California, and author of *The Foot Book,* dead skin houses fungi that can reinfect you. To remove it, use a bristled scrub brush on the entire foot and a baby bottle "nipple brush" on toe webs. And brush in the shower, so the dead skin goes down the drain without touching other parts of your body.

Be a shoe swapper. "In theory, you're supposed to wear a pair of shoes only once every five days in order to allow shoes to *really* dry out between wearings," adds Dr. Basler. "If people don't have enough shoes to do that, I suggest that they wear different pairs as often as possible."

High-powered help. The problem with over-the-counter medications is that the fungus often returns as soon as you stop using them. For serious bouts of athlete's foot, your doctor may recommend a prescription oral drug called griseofulvin, which knocks out the infection from the inside out.

Even with griseofulvin, however, you may need several months of treatment before your feet are clear again. "It's just not easy to knock out athlete's foot," says Ronald C. Savin, M.D., clinical professor of dermatology at Yale University School of Medicine in New Haven, Connecticut. "It often comes back, and we're not sure if that's because people catch it again or they really hadn't killed it in the first place."

BAD BREATH

Even with regular brushing and flossing, even with mints, mouthwashes and other breath fresheners, are there times when that h-h-h-horrendous h-h-h-halitosis h-h-h-has (*ugh!*) made some of those around you consider career opportunities in Arctic Circle weather stations?

If your mate or colleagues start inquiring about getting your mouth declared "endangered swamplands," don't take it *too* personally. After all, bad breath hits just about *everyone* sometime—and, unfortunately, everyone around them as well. "There are so many causes of bad breath, literally dozens of them, that it is occasionally difficult to pinpoint the cause," says Joseph Tonzetich, Ph.D., professor of oral biology at the University of British Columbia in Vancouver.

Fact is, just about anything you put in your mouth, from antihistamines and other drugs to food and drink, can make your breath smell a tad uglier. Stress, sinus problems, mouth sores, talking, even our hormones can intensify bad breath. But breathe easy, folks, because here's how to kiss that nasty halitosis goodbye.

Eat an orange. "Some cases of bad breath—particularly those caused by stress and taking drugs—are the result of your mouth being too dry," says Dr. Tonzetich. "Citrus fruits and other foods high in citric acids are very good at stimulating saliva. The acid also helps suppress the activity of some odor-causing enzymes, while the 'tangy' taste of lemons, oranges and grapefruit helps freshen your mouth."

Be a picker. "Probably one of the best ways to control bad breath is to use an oral irrigation device such as a Water Pik to 'irrigate' your teeth," says Fred G. Fedok, M.D., assistant professor of otolaryngology and head and neck surgery at University Hospital of Pennsylvania State University in Hershey. "Using a Water Pik helps remove food and other debris that cause a lot of bad breath."

Try the baking soda solution. You can add extra punch to your Water Pik by using a baking soda solution to clean your teeth. "You can brush on baking soda with a toothbrush and then rinse with water or use your Water Pik," says Dr. Fedok. "Or what I *really* recommend is mixing baking soda with warm water, pouring that solution into the Water Pik and using it to irrigate your teeth and mouth."

According to Dr. Fedok, "Baking soda is a great remedy for bad breath, because it changes the pH in your mouth and makes it a less friendly environment for many bacteria." He adds that baking soda is especially helpful to those with bad breath caused by gingivitis.

Brush your tongue. "Perhaps the most *overlooked* way of eliminating bad breath is to brush the top surface of the tongue when you brush your teeth," says Dr. Tonzetich. "Although there are many causes of bad breath, usually the odor arises from the surface of the tongue." That's because the tongue is covered with microscopic, hairlike projections that trap and harbor plaque and food, says Eric Shapira, D.D.S., assistant clinical professor and lecturer at the University of the Pacific School of Dentistry in San Francisco. A daily, gentle brushing (including the top of your tongue) unlodges these odorous particles.

Or give it a wipe. Don't have a toothbrush handy? Not to worry. "Simply take a hanky or a piece of gauze and give your tongue a good wiping," advises David S. Halpern, D.M.D., a dentist in Columbia, Maryland, and a spokesperson for the Academy of General Dentistry. "Even a quick wipe is good for re-moving the coating on your tongue that can cause bad breath."

Clean your sinuses. Since bad breath can be caused by any number of sinus problems, some people get relief by "washing" out the area inside the nose where the sinuses drain, says Dr. Fedok. If you want to try it, use a saline solution in a blue-ball syringe—the kind used to clean out ears. (Both the solu-tion and the syringe are available at most pharmacies.) "You'll have to refill the syringe several times. Spray the saline up each nostril, letting the solution drain out the other nostril and your mouth. It may take up to a pint of saline to wash out your sinuses," says Dr. Fedok.

Use the *right* mouthwash. Just about any type of mouthwash will temporarily mask the odors of bad breath—usually for about 20 minutes. But to eliminate the foul smell with the efficiency of Rambo in a bad mood, choose a mouthwash that contains zinc. "Zinc has a tendency to do a lot of things to inhibit the production of sulfur compounds that cause bad breath," says Dr. Tonzetich. "And zinc mouthwashes don't taste as metallic as copper-containing oral products."

Eat breakfast. Miss breakfast and it's a good bet you may have tainted breath *all* morning long, adds Dr. Tonzetich. "You usually have tainted breath until you take in some food," he says. "A lot of people who go without breakfast have bad breath at least until lunchtime."

Complete your dining with water. Whether you're having a quick snack or a multicourse meal, a water chaser is the ideal after-dining drink. "Swishing a mouthful of water is a great way to get rid of odors caused by food and drink," says Dr. Halpern. This is especially recommended after having coffee, tea, soft drinks or alcohol, which can leave a residue that can attach to plaque in your mouth, causing bad breath.

Settle your stomach. Indigestion or stomach problems can cause you to burp, expelling foul gaseous odors, says Dr. Halpern. To relieve this problem, take antacids to settle your stomach.

Don't dine with the garlic family. Highly spiced foods like to linger long after the party's over. Spices tend to stay and recirculate through essential oils they leave in your mouth. Depending on how much you eat, the odor can stay in your mouth up to 24 hours, no matter how often you brush your teeth. Some foods to avoid include onions, hot peppers and garlic.

Chew your "greens." Besides being instant breath fresheners, parsley and wintergreen also release pleasant aromatic substances into the lungs. The result: They'll be freshening your breath some 24 hours later, says Ronald S. Bogdasarian, M.D., an otorhino-laryngologist and clinical assistant professor at the University of Michigan School of Medicine in Ann Arbor who has done research into the causes and cures of bad breath.

Watch your diet. Some research indicates that a high-fat diet may contribute to bad breath. The theory is that certain fats—particularly those in cheeses, butter, whole milk and fatty meats—may contain certain aromatic substances that we metabolize and exhale, says Dr. Bogdasarian. If other causes of bad breath have been eliminated, try cutting back on deli meats and dairy products and replacing them with more carbohydrates, fruits, vegetables and whole grains.

Know your medications. Many prescription and over-the-counter drugs contribute to bad breath by having a "drying" effect on the mouth. That's because saliva, being slightly acidic, normally suppresses bacteria. But some drugs cause saliva to dry up. When it does, the bacteria in your mouth start reproducing like rabbits in springtime. Antihistamines, decongestants, anti-anxiety drugs, diuretics and certain heart medications lead the list of drugs that have a mouth-drying effect. If you're taking any of these drugs, be sure to *increase* your intake of water. Chewing gum or sucking on hard candies will also keep saliva flowing.

BELCHING

I n some parts of the world, the ultimate compliment you can pay the host after a hearty, sumptuous feast is one prolonged, expressive belch. That kind of complimentary noise won't earn you the Best Manners Award at Aunt Martha's Sunday buffet, but polite or not, belching *does* come naturally: A study has shown that healthy young people belch an average of 11 times in 20 hours—excluding mealtimes.

The gas you release while belching comes from your upper gastrointestinal tract. It got there because you swallowed it while talking, eating or drinking. The air that goes down with every swallow just adds to the air already in your stomach—and all this trapped air speaks loud and clear when it comes back up.

What to do when belching becomes a bother? Try these tips from our experts.

Eat modest meals at a measured pace. "Eat small meals, and eat slowly," advises Nicholas Talley, M.D., Ph.D., a gastroenterologist and associate professor of medicine at the Mayo Clinic in Rochester, Minnesota. Dr. Talley also recommends not eating and drinking at the same time to reduce repetitive swallowing.

Banish balloon food. Certain foods and beverages are particularly gassy or puffed up with air. Watch out for "carbonated or foaming beverages, or dishes made with beaten eggs or whipped cream," says Ronald L. Hoffman, M.D., director of the Hoffman Center for Holistic Medicine in New York City.

Break those air-grabbing habits. How else do you swallow air when you're not eating? According to Dr. Hoffman, smoking, sipping through a straw, chewing gum and sucking hard candies can add to the trapped air in your stomach and contribute to belching problems. Drinking from water fountains, cans and bottles can also be blamed. Try to avoid munching or chewing when you're on the go. And when you want a sip of something, try to drink calmly rather than grabbing a quick gulp.

Relax for relief. "Work to reduce your anxiety level," recommends Dr. Talley. "Sometimes you're swallowing air because you're anxious." Among the best stress relievers are regular exercise, meditation and soothing activities such as taking a hot bath.

Don't belch for relief. Many people don't realize that a forced belch will backfire, says Dr. Talley. When you try to force up the trapped air, he says, you often swallow more air at the time or just afterward, so you end up getting more air down than you actually remove. The bottom line: "Don't force yourself to belch," says Dr. Talley.

Do a trial run of antacids. Some people who feel they have excess stomach gas may benefit from over-the-counter antacids in standard doses, says Dr. Talley. That's because stomach acid sometimes reacts with food to create excess carbon dioxide in your stomach. If you do take antacids, begin with a short "trial run" to see whether they're effective, he suggests.

Forget the plop-plop-fizz-fizz. Effervescent over-the-counter remedies like Alka-Seltzer are no help to belchers, says Dr. Hoffman. Like carbonated beverages, these remedies make you belch even more, because you're swallowing more air along with the remedy.

Defoam those bubbles with simethicone. An ingredient in over-the-counter products like Maalox Plus and Mylanta, simethicone is a "defoaming" agent. "Simethicone works well for gas in the small intestine and reduces belching," Dr. Hoffman ·says. This belch blaster smashes up the biggest gas bubbles and breaks them into smaller ones that burst more easily.

Let your coffee cool a bit. "When you slurp a hot beverage, you swallow air," says Marvin L. Hanson, Ph.D., chairman of the Department of Communication Disorders at the University of Utah in Salt Lake City. To get around that problem, simply let your coffee cool a bit before you take a steamy sip.

BLEMISHES

You may have thought it was over, another chapter of adolescence that could be forgotten as easily as algebra or your high school gym teacher. But now, as you stare in the mirror at that huge red dot on your chin, you have more than memories to remind you of the bother of blemishes.

And you're not alone. Although considered to be primarily a torment of teenagers, blemishes continue to provide plenty of angst in adulthood, and they can occur in varying degrees of severity. Anyone with hormones can get blemishes—and of course, we've *all* got hormones.

"The severity of most blemishes is related to heredity, amount of oil secretion, hormones and, to some extent, stress," says Michael Ramsey, M.D., clinical instructor of dermatology at Baylor College of Medicine in Houston. But here's how you can put a quick end to your own private Zit Parade.

Don't scrub. The biggest mistake by the acne-prone is thinking that washing with might is washing right. "In fact, the friction you create by overscrubbing can stir up new blemishes and aggravate existing ones," says dermatologist Edward Bondi, M.D., who treats the acne-ridden at the University of Pennsylvania Hospital in Philadelphia. "You shouldn't even wash with a washcloth. Instead, gently clean your face with your hands."

Try medication. Use an over-the-counter medication with benzoyl peroxide. This active ingredient is "the first line of treatment and the best over-the-counter medication you can use," says Dr. Bondi. Oxy-5, Oxy-10, Fostex and Clearasil products are among those containing this active ingredient. But note that benzoyl peroxide is better at preventing new lesions than at getting rid of what you already have. "One common mistake is to dab it on the blemishes themselves," adds Dr. Bondi. "What's *more* effective is to spread it all over the face, especially in areas where acne is prone to be present."

Use it once a day at first, then as your face gets used to it, two or three times. Since you may not see improvements for six to eight weeks, try to be patient.

A prescription drug called tretinoin, a derivative of vitamin A, alters the growth of oil glands. Applied once a day, it can dry up current pimples and prevent others from forming. It may cause an uncomfortable burning or drying sensation, but most people soon get used to it, doctors say.

In a pinch, try calamine. If you feel a blemish flourishing and you're all out of benzoyl peroxide, there's no need to run to the all-night minimart. Calamine lotion absorbs excess skin oil and can help nip that blotch in the bud, advises Thomas Goodman, Jr., M.D., assistant professor of dermatology at the University of Tennessee Center for Health Sciences in Memphis.

Chill out to avoid blemishes. Controlling the stress in your life is one of the best ways to control acne and other blemishes. "There's no question that stress plays a key role in the development of new blemishes and continuance of existing ones," says Dr. Bondi. If you're prone to acne, find a relaxation technique that works for you—such as exercise, meditation or listening to music—and practice it daily, particularly when you're stressed out.

Put on a cube—cosmetically. Placing an ice cube on blemishes for about 60 seconds after washing can help make them less noticeable, because cold reduces inflammation, adds Dr. Goodman.

Get in the shade. Although sunshine tends to "camouflage" blemishes by tanning your hide, there's no scientific evidence that sunshine helps remedy pimples. And the sunlight may cause adverse skin reactions to some acne medications. If you notice your skin turning red and blotchy, "minimize exposure to sunlight, infrared heat lamps and even sunscreens," cautions Thomas Gossel, Ph.D., R.Ph., professor of pharmacology and toxicology and associate dean at Ohio Northern University College of Pharmacy in Ada and an expert on over-the-counter products.

Don't put too much hope in special soap. "Acne soaps tend to be very good at drying your skin, but many do *nothing* to treat acne," says Dr. Bondi. "Rather than buying a special 'acne' soap, you're better off getting the *right* soap for your skin." That means a gentle soap like Dove if you have dry skin—*especially* in the winter—and maybe a stronger soap if your skin is excessively oily.

Read the labels on your cosmetics. Oil-based makeups have long been known to trigger blemishes, because the oil is usually a derivative of fatty acids more potent than your body's acids.

"If you're prone to blemishes, you're better off with a makeup that lists water as one of its main ingredients," says Michael Stein, a Hollywood makeup artist whose company has touched up famous movie faces. Specific ingredients too rich for blemish-prone skin include lanolins, isopropyl myristate, laureth-4 and sodium lauryl sulfate.

Watch your diet. "Iodine *has* been associated with acne, so iodine-rich foods such as beef liver, clams, crabs and other shellfish should not be ingested in large quantities," says Dr. Ramsey. "And although scientific studies *haven't* shown that chocolate, sodas, greasy foods or milk aggravates acne, if you find that you break out after eating certain foods, then forget the studies and avoid those foods." Among the other likely suspects are cheeses, nuts and other high-fat foods, as well as caffeine.

BLISTERS

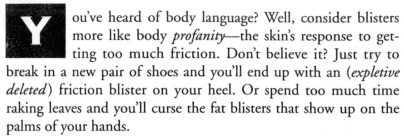

You've heard of body language? Well, consider blisters more like body *profanity*—the skin's response to getting too much friction. Don't believe it? Just try to break in a new pair of shoes and you'll end up with an (*expletive deleted*) friction blister on your heel. Or spend too much time raking leaves and you'll curse the fat blisters that show up on the palms of your hands.

But since there will always be new shoes to break in and lawns in need of care, there will always be blisters—*unless* you take some precautions. So here's how to banish that blister before it articulates new meanings for the nastiest four-letter word of all—*pain*. Let's start with the most prevalent kind—foot blisters.

Give your feet a lube job. "Blisters are the result of too much friction. To avoid some of that friction and prevent a blister, liberally rub Vaseline over your feet," says Robert Diamond, D.P.M., a Pennsylvania podiatrist affiliated with Muhlenberg Hospital Center in Bethlehem and Allentown Osteopathic Hospital. "If the shoe doesn't fit correctly and your foot is slipping, you'll have better glide, so there's less friction—and therefore less chance of developing a friction blister."

Quit the cotton. Sorry, but much-ballyhooed cotton sweat socks *don't* offer the best protection against blisters. In fact, sports podiatrists say that man-made acrylic socks are best for preventing blisters. "Cotton fiber becomes abrasive with repeated use, and it also compresses and loses its shape and 'cushion' when wet," says Douglas Richie, Jr., D.P.M., clinical instructor of podiatry at Los Angeles County–University of Southern California Medical Center in Los Angeles. According to Dr. Richie, "The shape of the sock is critical when it's inside a shoe." So a sock that loses its shape is just what your blister-vulnerable foot *doesn't* need.

Silken your skin. "Wearing a silk undersock can help prevent foot blisters and relieve the pain once you get them, since silk is less damaging to the skin than other fabrics," says Nicholas J. Lowe, M.D., clinical professor of dermatology at the University of California, Los Angeles, School of Medicine and director of the Skin Research Foundation of California in Santa Monica.

Use powder power. Rubbing baby powder on your feet *before* any blister-promoting activity is another good preventer. "Make powdering part of your daily routine," says Richard Cowin, D.P.M., director of Cowin Foot Clinic of Orlando, Florida. Reason: Like petroleum jelly, it helps reduce friction and eases glide.

Put new footwear in your handbag. "Probably the biggest cause of foot blisters in women comes from trying to break in a new pair of shoes," says dermatologist Joseph Bark, M.D., past chairman of the Department of Dermatology at St. Joseph's Hospital in Lexington, Kentucky. "My advice to women who get a new pair of shoes? Wear them for only 30 minutes at a time. It's all right to wear the shoes several times a day, but only for 30 minutes—at least for the first few days." (So carry an extra pair of broken-in shoes in your handbag and trade off a few times during the day.)

Pad it with moleskin. A moleskin pad (available at most drugstores) is the best preventive measure for the blister-prone, and it's also great for *relieving* pain once the blister forms. Cut the moleskin into a doughnut shape and place it over the blister (or the area where you're prone to get it). "Leave the central area open over the blister," advises Suzanne Tanner, M.D., assistant professor of orthopedics at the University of Colorado Sportsmedicine Center in Denver. The surrounding moleskin will absorb the shock and friction that cause or aggravate blisters.

Try a heel lift. Blisters on the back of the foot? They could be blamed on the heel counter—the tough shoe leather that covers your heel. If the counter rubs the wrong area of your foot, you'll have blister trouble fast. The fix? "All you usually have to do is put in a heel lift," says Dr. Cowin. Make sure to use the same size heel lift in *both* shoes unless advised differently by your doctor, even if only one heel is blistering.

Use an insole. To avoid blisters on the heel and other parts of the foot, many doctors recommend a Spenco insole. These store-bought inserts cut down on friction to prevent new blisters and help ease the pain of existing ones, says Dr. Diamond.

Soak 'em in Epsom. "If you perspire too much, you're more prone to getting blisters," adds Dr. Diamond. "If that's your problem, soaking feet in Epsom salts can help dry excessive sweating." Dissolve Epsom salts in warm water and soak your feet for about five minutes at the end of the day. Then dry thoroughly.

Give a double dose of healing gel. Research shows that triple antibiotic ointments can eliminate bacterial contamination after *two* applications. Neosporin and other nonprescription antibiotic ointments are sold in all drugstores. Avoid old standbys such as iodine and camphor-phenol, because they delay healing. After applying the antibiotic, you should cover the area with a gauze pad—but change that covering each time it gets wet to avoid contamination.

For hands—try a combination play. If your problem is hand blisters rather than foot blisters, the Epsom salts relief can be a big help. Also, wear heavy-duty work gloves whenever you have yard work to do. Another way to prevent blisters on your hands: Follow the advice of Dr. Cowin and rub some baby powder on your hands.

BLOODSHOT EYES

Party into the wee hours of the morning and the town isn't the only thing that will be painted red: Don't be surprised if your morning-after eyes resemble a ruby-colored road map.

Of course, heavy partying is not the only way to make your eyes burn red the next morning. Colds, allergies, even swimming in a chlorinated pool turns eyes bloodshot. But rest assured, the damage is usually minor and temporary. Here's how to whiten up those eyes again.

Apply a cold compress. If your eyes itch, the bloodshot look is probably caused by allergies. "A cold washcloth placed over your eyes will soothe the pain and shrink the blood vessels if your eyes are bloodshot because of allergies," says Eric Donnenfeld, M.D., associate professor of ophthalmology at North Shore University Hospital–Cornell Medical College in Manhasset, New York. Hold the cold compress over your eyes until the itchiness subsides. You can repeat as often as convenient during the day.

For tired eyes—use a warm compress. If your eyes are red but don't itch, then a warm compress is the answer, adds Dr. Donnenfeld: "Warmth is best for bloodshot eyes caused by fatigue, staying up too late or a cold." Just place a warm washcloth over your closed eyes for 10 to 20 minutes.

Try artificial tears. If your bloodshot eyes are stinging, try soothing them with preservative-free artificial tears, suggests Paul Vinger, M.D., assistant clinical professor of ophthalmology at Harvard University in Cambridge, Massachusetts. He recommends the single-dose packages.

Contacts wearers: Read the label. If you're a contact lens wearer and you notice more eye redness than in the past, read the label on your contact lens cleaner. If you're not using one labeled "preservative-free," switch to one that is.

LOOK FOR THE
RED BADGE OF AGING

There's a patch of blood in the white of your eye, and you can't remember anything happening. There's no swelling, no pain, no loss of vision, nothing. Just a blotch of red.

If that's the case, then relax. "It's a common occurrence, especially if you're over 40," says Michael Marmor, M.D., an ophthalmologist and chairman of the Department of Ophthalmology at Stanford University Medical Center in California. "The blood will go away by itself. You can't do anything for it. Eyedrops won't do any good. It will go away by itself in one to two weeks. The hardest part of the whole thing will be trying to think up a story to explain to your friends how it happened."

Put a lid on "red-out" products. "Eyedrops that promise to remove redness should be used only occasionally, because they can become habit forming," warns Dr. Donnenfeld. "After using them for a while, you may develop a 'rebound' effect, so if you *don't* use the drops, your eyes become red." His advice: Avoid using these over-the-counter products for more than four consecutive days, and try not to use them more than once daily.

Avoid known allergens. Steer clear of anything that has caused you to have allergies in the past: It could be causing your red-eye to flare up. In addition, wash your hands after touching pets or applying makeup and shampoo, advises Thomas Platts-Mills, M.D., Ph.D., head of the Division of Allergy and Clinical Immunology at the University of Virginia Health Sciences Center in Charlottesville.

BODY ODOR

Back when our ancestors were walking on their knuckles, when there were no Johnny Mathis records or candlelight dinners to help set the mood, most folks had a nice, natural ripeness that may have turned on their dinner companions more than it turned them off.

How times change. These days, that same natural body odor can leave you lonelier than ol' Uncle Ugh before his end-of-month bath night. Of course, the smell-good departments of pharmacies and supermarkets are well stocked with a scented array of deodorants, which kill the bacteria that cause the odor or mask the smell that the bacteria create, but many people get irritations from deodorants and antiperspirants. There *are* other ways to banish body odor—sans deodorant—and here are some of the most effective.

Don't stink with zinc. Some people find that body odor problems can be remedied simply by consuming more zinc, says Morton Scribner, M.D., a dermatologist in Arcadia, California. He suggests that you boost intake with a daily supplement of 25 to 50 milligrams of zinc. Or steer toward zinc-rich foods such as oysters, lean beef, king crab and wheat germ.

"Roll on" some baking soda. "Sodium bicarbonate, better known as baking soda, kills the odor-causing bacteria and absorbs moisture," says Arthur Jacknowitz, Pharm.D., professor and chairman of clinical pharmacy at West Virginia University School of Pharmacy in Morgantown. "Many people find that baking soda is just as effective as a deodorant." Simply sprinkle a generous amount into your bath and soak yourself, or mix it with a little talcum powder and apply it directly to underarms.

Clean yourself the way doctors do. Surgeons scrub with antibacterial soap before an operation in order to kill bacteria. These soaps are "great for people with problem body odor or a tendency to get irritated from deodorants," says John F. Romano, M.D., a dermatologist and clinical assistant professor of medicine at The New York Hospital—Cornell Medical Center in New York City. And they're available over the counter at most drugstores. "Just ask the pharmacist for a surgical 'scrub' soap, then wash with it to kill the bacteria that cause body odors," says Dr. Romano. Scrub soap is very effective, yet gentle enough to use in the groin and underarm areas, he adds.

Do don some Domeboro. Another over-the-counter product that's an effective alternative to deodorant is Domeboro, according to D'Anne Kleinsmith, M.D., a cosmetic dermatologist at William Beaumont Hospital near Detroit. Domeboro is a powder that you mix in cool or lukewarm water and apply to your problem areas. "It will relieve odor and wetness in those areas— whether it's your underarms, groin or feet or under your breasts," says Dr. Kleinsmith.

Hold the spices. Extracts of proteins and oils from certain foods and spices remain in your body's excretions and secretions for hours after you eat them. These extracts can impart an odor. Fish, cumin, curry and garlic lead the list. "So if you have body odor problems, you'll have *more* problems if you eat a lot of these foods," says Dr. Kleinsmith.

Take a walk on the wild side. Forget the latest perfumes from Paris. Hunters have a way of coming up with their own fragrances. The name of the game in hunting, according to some, is to mask all trace of body odor lest the deer or bear being stalked catches wind of trouble and flees for cover.

How do hunters do it? One popular odor mask is pine soap, available in most hunting supply stores, says Dave Petzal, a veteran hunter and the executive editor of *Field and Stream* magazine. Pine soap not only masks human odor but "leaves you smelling like a pine forest," he says. If pine forest isn't your style, some hunters are using plain old glycerin soap.

CHAFING

Now here's a condition that really rubs you the wrong way. You buy a wash-and-wear outfit to make your life a little easier, or you decide to get your body into shape with a new exercise program—and what happens? Your skin gets all irritated and sore.

Mild chafing happens to everyone, and usually just applying baby powder or talc to the problem area will help keep your skin happy. Another easy prevention technique is to wear a soft fabric like cotton rather than a more abrasive synthetic blend or a rough wool. But if your hide can't seem to hide from chafing, here's what to do.

Zap it with zinc. "Zinc oxide, the white paste that life-guards put on their noses, is wonderful for treating chafing—it's simple and inexpensive," says dermatologist John F. Romano, M.D., clinical assistant professor of medicine at The New York Hospital–Cornell Medical Center in New York City. "Just apply a thin layer on the area where you tend to chafe. If you have trouble removing the zinc oxide because that area is hairy, apply a little olive oil or mineral oil and wipe it off."

Smear on petroleum jelly. Another simple and inexpensive remedy is petroleum jelly. "It's best to apply the jelly before you exercise," says D'Anne Kleinsmith, M.D., a cosmetic dermatologist at William Beaumont Hospital near Detroit. The petroleum jelly protects the area from friction.

And there might be some areas that need special attention. "Runners frequently complain that their nipples get chafed by a shirt in the up-and-down motion. I advise my patients to spread some petroleum jelly over their nipples before running," says Dr. Kleinsmith. For even more protection, cover each nipple with a small adhesive bandage.

Put away the panty hose. Women who are prone to chafing should definitely avoid wearing panty hose, according to

Dr. Kleinsmith. "Panty hose don't allow the skin in your upper thighs to breathe," she says.

Keep it tight. A pair of the electric-colored, stretchy-fabric athletic tights or Lycra cycling shorts may be ideal because they are snug, yet stretch, and cause no friction against the skin, says Tom Barringer, M.D., a family physician in Charlotte, North Carolina, who is a fitness runner.

Men: Switch to boxers. Men who get chafing around the waist, crotch and upper thighs might want to try wearing boxer shorts. Tighter-fitting jockey underwear is more likely to cause chafing around the waist and thighs.

Wash before you wear. Be sure to wash any new clothes before you wear them, says Richard H. Strauss, M.D., a sports medicine doctor at Ohio State University College of Medicine in Columbus. Washing sometimes softens fabric enough to lessen abrasion. It also removes dyes and sizing (chemicals used to add crispness and luster to new clothes) that can irritate skin in some people, says Dr. Romano. Washing is especially important when you wear dyed exercise clothes, he adds. The skin absorbs dye as you sweat—and that's something you want to avoid.

Wrap it up. People who are overweight or who have big thighs are more likely to have chafing, but there's an easy way to find relief. Wrap elastic bandages around the portions of the legs that rub, suggests Dr. Barringer. For any vigorous exercise, wrap elastic bandages around each thigh or wear cycling-style shorts, which come down farther on the thigh and are tighter than regular shorts. That will shield the skin on the inside of your thighs. But be sure the elastic bandage is secure, so it does not move across the skin.

CHAPPED LIPS

As if squeezing down chimney after chimney with a 46-inch waist isn't impressive enough, what's truly amazing about Santa is how he manages to grin merrily all winter long. After all, when the rest of us try to crack a smile during the Yule season, we literally *crack* a smile—courtesy of chapped lips.

Unlike your skin, lips lack the natural oils needed to protect against drying winter winds and the low humidity of indoor heating. And lips are easily burned by the sun's rays (which do double damage when reflecting off snow) because they contain no melanin, the pigment in the rest of the skin that causes freckles and suntan. But here's how to give the kiss-off to chapped lips and smile without wincing through those dry winter months.

Don't lick the problem. Since chapped lips are *dry* lips, the obvious answer is to simply lick your lips to keep them moist, right?

Wrong: "This is one of the very *worst* things people can do," says Ronald Sherman, M.D., a dermatologist and member of the attending staff at Mount Sinai Medical Center in New York City. "It only *increases* chapping. When the moisture from licking your lips evaporates, so does some of the moisture from your lips." Another problem is that lip lickers tend to also be lip biters, and biting your lips removes the protective layer of skin.

Water your dry cells. Drinking additional fluids in the winter is a natural and easy way to keep your lips from chapping. "I recommend several ounces of water every few hours," says Diana Bihova, M.D., clinical assistant professor of dermatology at New York University Medical Center in New York City. "As you age, the ability of your cells to retain moisture decreases, so your dryness problem may actually increase each winter. Another way to help counter wintertime dry lips is to humidify the air in your home and office."

Be wise to vitamin B. "Nutritional deficiencies—such as the lack of B-complex vitamins and iron—can play a part in scaling of the lips and cracking at the corners of the mouth," says Nelson Lee Novick, M.D., associate clinical professor of dermatology at Mount Sinai School of Medicine in New York City. "So make sure you're okay on that front with a multivitamin/mineral supplement."

Apply lip balm frequently. "You should apply lip balm every hour or two—both to prevent chapped lips and to treat them once you get them," says John F. Romano, M.D., a dermatologist and clinical assistant professor of medicine at The New York Hospital–Cornell Medical Center in New York City.

Using petroleum jelly is fine, but if you go with a commercial product specifically made for chapped lips, "make sure you use one that contains sunscreen with an SPF [sun protection factor] of at least 15," adds Nicholas J. Lowe, M.D., clinical professor of dermatology at the University of California, Los Angeles, School of Medicine and director of the Skin Research Foundation of California in Santa Monica.

Mind your own beeswax. "To my mind, the single best product for chapped lips is Carmex. It's an old-fashioned product that comes in a little tin and contains, among other things, beeswax and phenol," offers Rodney Basler, M.D., assistant professor of internal medicine at the University of Nebraska Medical Center in Omaha. "I'd say no prescription medication is better than that."

Give toothpaste the brush-off. "Allergy and sensitivity to flavoring agents in toothpaste, candy, chewing gum and mouthwash can cause chapped lips in some people," says Thomas Goodman, Jr., M.D., assistant professor of dermatology at the University of Tennessee Center for Health Sciences in Memphis. "Cinnamon-flavored products and some tartar control toothpastes can be especially irritating. I tell my patients to avoid them."

CONSTIPATION

What goes up must come down. Sir Isaac Newton proved that, sitting under an apple tree.

What goes in must come out. You proved that, sitting on the toilet this morning.

Well, *didn't* you?

Or was it yesterday morning that you had your last bowel movement? Or the day before? Or one cold but memorable day early last December?

Constipation is no fun. Sometimes it can be painful. But the cause of your sluggish bowels is often easy to find. It may include a lack of fiber in the diet, insufficient liquid intake, stress, medications, lack of exercise and bad bowel habits, says Paul Rousseau, M.D., chief of the Department of Geriatrics at the Carl T. Hayden Veterans Administration Medical Center in Phoenix, Arizona.

We take a look at all of these factors, and ways to remedy the situation below.

Lotion the motion with fiber. "Go on a high-fiber diet," says Edward P. Donatelle, M.D., professor emeritus of the Department of Family Practice and Community Medicine at the University of Kansas School of Medicine in Wichita. Soluble fiber, found in grains, legumes and fruits, is particularly effective. Oatmeal, rice, wheat germ, corn bran, prunes, raisins, apricots, figs and an apple a day are all good sources, Dr. Donatelle says.

Try a natural laxative. For a concentrated constipation buster, go for a fiber supplement that will budge that balky bowel. One of the best is psyllium, which is sold in health food stores. Marvin M. Schuster, M.D., chief of the Department of Digestive Diseases at Francis Scott Key Medical Center in Baltimore, recommends one teaspoon of psyllium with meals. Add the teaspoonful to a glass of water or juice and stir thoroughly before drinking. (You can also make a "paste" of one teaspoon of psyllium moistened with water, but be sure to drink at least a full glass of juice or water afterward.) Another alternative: Metamucil, a bowel regulator that contains psyllium and is sold in most drugstores and some supermarkets.

Use fluids to fuel the fiber. "Drink plenty of fluids," says John Sutherland, M.D., clinical professor of family practice at the University of Iowa College of Medicine in Iowa City and director of the Waterloo Family Practice Residency Program in Waterloo. Fluid expands and softens the fiber you're eating, allowing it to form bulk in the colon. That bulking action in turn triggers the urge to move your bowels.

"Ordinarily, you need to drink about a gallon of fluid a day—the more, the better," Dr. Sutherland says.

Avoid milk and cheese. If you have a problem with constipation, try avoiding milk products temporarily, says Dr. Donatelle. Both milk and cheese contain casein, an insoluble protein that tends to plug up the intestinal tract.

Get your body moving and your bowels will, too. "Exercise can help that lazy bowel to function better," says gastroenterologist Nicholas Talley, M.D., Ph.D., associate professor of medicine at the Mayo Clinic in Rochester, Minnesota. "Aerobic exercise such as walking, running and swimming is best." If you're a walker, for instance, go for a brisk 20- to 30-minute arm-swinging stroll every day.

Listen when your body talks. "Sometimes people who are constipated ignore 'the urge' and wait until later. This can aggravate the problem," says Dr. Sutherland. When your body tells you it's time to go, head for the bathroom as soon as possible.

Get into training. You can actually train your bowels to get on a regular schedule, says Vera Loening-Baucke, M.D., a pediatrician at the University of Iowa Hospitals and Clinics in Iowa City. Her advice: Sit on the toilet for about ten minutes after the same meal every day. The key is to stay relaxed. Eventually, says Dr. Loening-Baucke, your body will catch on.

BE SELECTIVE ABOUT LAXATIVES

Many over-the-counter products are sold as laxatives, but not all laxatives are recommended by doctors. In fact, heavy use of some laxatives can be counterproductive and even risky, according to Ronald L. Hoffman, M.D., director of the Hoffman Center for Holistic Medicine in New York City.

Heavy use of some laxatives can give you diarrhea, according to Dr. Hoffman. And many are habit-forming: If you always rely on a laxative to prompt bowel movements, your body may begin to need it to trigger the action. Laxatives containing castor oil can damage your intestinal lining, and those that have mineral oil can interfere with your ability to absorb certain vitamins and minerals, according to Dr. Hoffman.

Safest are the natural or vegetable laxative products, high-fiber bulking agents such as Metamucil, Citrucel or Perdiem that are sold in most drugstores. "If you can't tolerate a high-fiber diet, these bulking agents are very safe, helpful supplements," according to gastroenterologist Nicholas Talley, M.D., Ph.D., associate professor of medicine at the Mayo Clinic in Rochester, Minnesota.

Dr. Talley recommends taking the cautious approach with bulking agents. Follow the directions on the package, increasing the dosage slowly if needed.

Reach for the rhubarb. "When it's in season in early summer, fresh rhubarb is a delicious and powerful antidote to constipation," says Ronald L. Hoffman, M.D., director of the Hoffman Center for Holistic Medicine in New York City. It contains a good amount of fiber, which helps keep things moving.

For a rhubarb juice refresher that will get your tract on track, try this cooling recipe: Chop three stalks of rhubarb (remove the leaves, which are toxic) and mix with one cup of apple juice, ¼ of a peeled lemon and one teaspoon of honey. Put all the ingredients in a blender or food processor and puree until smooth.

Some advice: Try a small amount of rhubarb juice at first and see how your body responds. It can be as powerful and quick-acting as prune juice. Also, depending on how you like the taste, you might want to mix it with other juices. *Caution:* Rhubarb should be avoided by people with a history of calcium kidney stones.

Don't strain. As tempting as it may be to huff and puff your way out of constipation, it is not wise to do so. You risk giving yourself hemorrhoids and anal fissures, which not only are painful, but can also aggravate your constipation by narrowing the anal opening. Straining can also raise your blood pressure and lower your heartbeat. Dr. Rousseau says he has known several elderly patients to black out and fall off the toilet, sometimes suffering fractures as a result—which brings us back once again to Sir Isaac Newton and those immutable laws of gravity.

Review your Rx. Medicines that can contribute to constipation include prescription antidepressants and painkillers as well as some over-the-counter remedies such as iron supplements and aluminum-containing antacids. Dr. Hoffman recommends that you check with your doctor if you suspect your medication is causing your constipation.

CONTACT LENS PROBLEMS

The disposable contact lens has joined the Q-Tip as a personal care item with a very short life. But don't think disposable contact lenses (or any other type) are worry-free just because they're so convenient. Eye doctors say *any* lens can become contaminated and cause eye damage. Here's how to see your way to eye health.

To be safe, avoid sleeping with lenses in. Even if you have contact lenses that are labeled "extended wear," it doesn't mean you should leave them in every night. According to a study at the Massachusetts Eye and Ear Infirmary and Harvard Medical School in Boston, you raise your risk of ulceration 5 percent for each night you sleep with extended-wear lenses in. The reason: Continuously worn contacts rub away the cornea (the covering of the eyeball). This causes tiny rips that invite infection and may lead to vision loss. Also, covering the cornea for extended periods blocks out oxygen, providing an ideal breeding ground for harmful bacteria. "My recommendation is to never sleep wearing any lenses, period," says Mitchell H. Friedlaender, M.D., director of the Cornea Service at the Scripps Clinic and Research Foundation in La Jolla, California.

Clean and disinfect any time you remove lenses. Whenever you take out your lenses, they must be cleaned as well as disinfected, says Joseph P. Shovlin, O.D., an optometrist at the Northeastern Eye Institute, with headquarters in Scranton, Pennsylvania, and chairman of the Contact Lens Section of the American Optometric Association. And if you wear the disposable kind, be sure to throw them away at the time prescribed by your doctor.

Clean the lens case, too. Scrub the case with hot water every other day with a toothbrush that's used only for that purpose, says Dr. Friedlaender.

Never use homemade saline solutions. Use a fresh solution each day, and use only commercial contact lens preparations. That's because homemade salt solutions might harbor a microorganism that can scar the cornea and cause partial or complete blindness, according to studies at the Centers for Disease Control and Prevention in Atlanta. And since tap water, distilled water and mineral water are not sterile, they may harbor infection-causing impurities, says Dr. Friedlaender. "Don't use them with contacts."

Stick with one lens-care regimen. A disinfecting/cleaning regimen is always specified for your lens type, says Thomas Gossel, Ph.D., R.Ph., professor of pharmacology and toxicology, and associate dean at Ohio Northern University College of Pharmacy in Ada. And that shouldn't be changed. If you switch from chemical to heat, for example, chemicals might be "baked into" soft lenses, and that could irritate your eyes. Whatever the recommended procedure, be sure to stick with it!

Never lick your lenses. Saliva is teeming with bacteria. "If you give your lenses a spit bath, you might as well rub your lenses on the floor," says Dr. Friedlaender.

Makeup first, lenses second. Use water-based, not oil-based, cosmetics, says Dr. Friedlaender, and apply makeup and hair spray before you put in your lenses. Around the eyes, use water-resistant mascara and apply to lash tips only, he adds.

Take out your lenses before swimming. The risk of wearing hard lenses in a pool or tub is that they may float out if your eyes get wet. With soft lenses, impurities in the water might be absorbed, which could cause infection, according to Paul Vinger, M.D., assistant clinical professor of ophthalmology at Harvard University in Cambridge, Massachusetts. "If you need to see underwater, get prescription goggles," says Dr. Vinger.

Switch to glasses before that big cleaning job. Remove contacts when using volatile household cleaners, which

HANDLE WITH CARE

C ontact lenses can be more than irritating. They also can be a breeding ground for pseudomonas bacteria. "It's not very fastidious—it can grow in anything moist and does very well in contact lens cases. And people who wear the extended-wear lenses have a ten times higher risk than daily lens wearers," says Gilbert Smolin, M.D., clinical professor of ophthalmology at the University of California, San Francisco, and research ophthalmologist at the Proctor Foundation, which specializes in external and infectious eye diseases.

The infections usually start off slowly without severe symptoms, Dr. Smolin says. "But the organism grows at a tremendously rapid rate," he says. "In severe infections, we've seen patients come in holding their hands under their eyes to catch the pus. Pseudomonas is particularly virulent—it can even cause loss of the eye—but it's not very contagious."

The treatment is "a very high dose of antibiotic drops as soon as possible," says Dr. Smolin. The infection generally clears up in a few days, but severe cases can take weeks. Fortunately, this condition is highly preventable. All it requires is good hygiene when it comes to caring for your contact lenses.

may be absorbed by the lenses, advises Scott MacRae, M.D., associate professor of ophthalmology at Oregon Health Sciences University in Portland and chairman of the Public Health Committee of the American Academy of Ophthalmology. "Volatile" cleaners include any cleaner containing ammonia or another strong-smelling chemical.

Remove your contacts if your eyes turn red. If your eyes become irritated, remove your contacts, says Dr. Shovlin. If the irritation doesn't go away after two to three hours, contact your eye-care practitioner. Tears, discharge, redness around the eyes and a change in vision are all indications of eye irritation.

CYSTS

Sometimes unpleasant things just happen without any reason. You get caught in a downpour without an umbrella. You get a flat tire on the way to the airport. You spill ketchup on your suit a few minutes before an important meeting. Or you get a cyst.

In a world of random events, getting a cyst is right up there with the least of the least explainable. Doctors don't know for certain how or why they develop.

Cysts are permanent little lumps, usually harmless and almost always painless, that can appear anywhere on your body but especially around the head, neck and back. The surface of a cyst is smooth, but underneath there's some problem that causes the swelling—a buildup of the body's natural oil (sebum), layers of impacted hair follicles or layers of accumulated skin scales.

Usually it's no big deal. You might see an enlarged, dark pore on the surface, and sometimes there's a bit of oozing. With doctor-prescribed medications and some surgical procedures, a cyst can be treated or removed. But as long as the cyst is not infected and doesn't burst, you can usually just live with it. In fact, the leading advice from dermatologists is:

Let it be. "If the cyst is small and unobtrusive, if it doesn't hurt or itch and if it isn't red or tender, then you can just leave it alone," says Jack L. Lesher, Jr., M.D., associate professor of dermatology at the Medical College of Georgia in Augusta. A hands-off policy is best for any cyst. Don't touch, pick, paw, squeeze or manipulate it in any way. If the cyst is in a position where it can easily be bumped or scratched, shield it with a gauze pad or some moleskin.

Apply warm compresses. Is the cyst red, oozing its contents or just plain sore? Place a washcloth soaked in warm (not hot) water over the irritated cyst several times a day, says Loretta S. Davis, M.D., assistant professor of dermatology at the Medical College of Georgia in Augusta. "This will increase the blood circulation to the area, quieting down an angry cyst."

LOWER THE CYST RISKS

Any unusual growth or mark on your skin that you're not sure about should be checked by your doctor. It could be cancerous. And even a benign cyst can warrant special medical attention.

"If a cyst appears to be growing, if it hurts or itches or if it's swollen and oozing profusely, it may be showing signs of serious infection," says Jack L. Lesher, Jr., M.D., associate professor of dermatology at the Medical College of Georgia in Augusta. "You'll need to see a dermatologist to have the cyst surgically removed or treated with antibiotics."

There's also a chance of severe infection after a cyst bursts or ruptures, so be sure to see the doctor if this occurs.

Wash and dress a ruptured cyst. "If a cyst should rupture and drain, you run the risk of developing a severe infection," says dermatologist Joseph Bark, M.D., past chairman of the Department of Dermatology at St. Joseph's Hospital in Lexington, Kentucky. "Wash it with soap and water, dab on some hydrogen peroxide with a cotton ball, and apply an antibacterial ointment such as Polysporin. Cover the area with a bandage or gauze pad to keep dirt off it until a doctor can check it out."

Never, ever remove a cyst yourself. "Bathroom surgery is the worst thing you can do for a cyst," says Dr. Davis. "If you squeeze it, some of the contents will probably be forced deeper into the skin. Your body will view it as foreign material and react with an extreme inflammation. Infection may also occur. You'll succeed only in turning a quiet cyst into an angry one, as well as in leaving a scar."

DANDRUFF

Everyone has dandruff—at least *some* dandruff—and that includes bald people. That's because every human scalp sheds dead cells, which "flake" off as new ones are pushed up from deeper skin layers. When these flakes become obvious on our hair and clothing, we call them dandruff. Perfectly natural stuff—but too often, we're made to feel as though this "problem" falls somewhere between global warming and playing high-stakes poker with someone named Ace.

In reality, there's nothing unusual about dandruff, and it definitely *doesn't* mean you're going bald. But here's how to remedy this nuisance if you're itching for some answers.

Lather twice. Always lather twice with a dandruff shampoo, says R. Jeffrey Herten, M.D., assistant clinical professor of dermatology at the University of California, Irvine, California College of Medicine. Work up the first lather as soon as you step into the shower so the shampoo has sufficient time to work. Leave it on until you're just about finished with your shower. Then rinse your hair very thoroughly. Follow that with a quick second lather and rinse. The second rinse will leave just a bit of the medication on your scalp so it can work until your next shampoo.

Hit the showers. If you ignore dandruff or the flakiness associated with the use of hair cosmetics, you allow scale to build, resulting in itchiness and possible infection, says Maria Hordinsky, M.D., associate professor of dermatology at the University of Minnesota Medical School in Minneapolis and the director of the Center for Hair Diseases at the University of Minnesota. Most experts say that shampooing often—daily, if necessary—with a specially medicated "dandruff" shampoo is the best way to control this problem.

Spread some oil. "Massaging some heated pure virgin olive oil into the scalp and then vigorously brushing with a natural-bristle hairbrush helps loosen dandruff scales," says Markus

Bluestein, a St. Louis hair stylist and makeup consultant. "It's also an excellent way to treat a dry scalp—the cause of much of the flaky, 'snowy' dandruff. You should microwave the oil until it's warm to the touch and apply it no more than twice a week. Each time, leave it on for about 20 minutes and then wash it out with a good shampoo."

Beat the tar out of it. If too much oil is your problem, you'll see "chunkier" dandruff that looks greasy and has a yellowish tint. Go with a tar-based shampoo such as Ionil T or Neutrogena's T/Gel. If you have blond or graying hair, however, stay away from tar shampoos, because they can give your hair a brownish tint, warns Patricia Farris, M.D., a dermatologist and clinical assistant professor at Tulane University School of Medicine in New Orleans.

Invest extra thyme. A potion made with thyme is believed to have medicinal powers that help dandruff when the solution is rinsed into the hair after shampooing, says New York City hair stylist Louis Gignac, owner of Louis-Guy D Salon and author of *Everything You Need to Know to Have Great-Looking Hair*. Boil four heaping tablespoons of dried thyme in two cups of water for ten minutes. Strain it and allow the brew to cool. Then pour half over your just-shampooed hair while it's still damp. Massage in gently and *don't* rinse. (Store the rest in the refrigerator for another treatment.)

DENTURE PROBLEMS

Everyone knows George Washington sported a set of dentures. But did you know that troublesome tusks ruined a world cruise for President Ulysses S. Grant? The bearded president, perhaps while admiring the whitecaps, leaned over the rail and, oops, down went his dentures into the briny deep.

You have to pity those poor denture wearers of yesterday. Before the age of super-sticky denture creams and pastes, artificial teeth were so loose many people removed them while they were eating.

Thank goodness things have changed. Or have they? If you're wearing a new set of dentures, you may be wrestling with some of the age-old problems: sore mouth, difficulty in eating or talking, dentures that slip and a feeling that perhaps they just don't look real.

Today, denture wearers have several choices of dental ware. There are partial and full dentures, those that can be removed and those that are implanted into the bone and become like real teeth.

All of them, like any artificial body part, take some getting used to, says prosthodontist George A. Murrell, D.D.S., of Manhattan Beach, California, who teaches at the University of Southern California School of Dentistry, Los Angeles. He and other specialists have some suggestions.

Steam your vegetables. "You tend to bite your cheek or tongue when you get a new set of dentures—particularly your first set," says Frank Wiebelt, D.D.S., associate professor and chairman of the Department of Removable Prosthodontics at the College of Dentistry at the University of Oklahoma Health Sciences Center in Oklahoma City. To avoid this, chew slowly. Also, stay away from raw vegetables or anything else that's crunchy or difficult to chew. "It's funny, because one of the first things my patients want to eat when they get new dentures is a steak and a salad, and both are among the most difficult things to eat," he says. "A steak is very tough. And believe it or not, lettuce is also difficult to chew. So eat your vegetables, but eat them steamed, and try to avoid anything that's tough for the first two weeks or so."

ARE YOUR DENTURES THE RIGHT FIT?

I t takes more than a month for most people to adjust to new dentures. But don't wait that long if you notice any of these symptoms, which can indicate a problem in the fit of your set.

- Teeth don't meet properly. "When you close your mouth, the top and bottom dentures should meet at both sides of your mouth," says Frank Wiebelt, D.D.S., associate professor and chairman of the Department of Removable Prosthodontics at the College of Dentistry at the University of Oklahoma Health Sciences Center in Oklahoma City. "If they meet only on one side, that's one sign the fit is wrong."
- The denture "teeth" are too long, resulting in problems with closing your mouth. (Your dentist can simply file down the teeth that are too long.)
- Dentures continually cut into your gums or cheeks.

Read out loud. New dentures can make talking difficult for the first week or so. One of the best ways to overcome this problem is to read out loud, advises Jerry F. Taintor, D.D.S., an endodontist in Memphis, Tennessee. As you're reading, listen to your pronunciation and your diction and correct what doesn't sound right.

"Keep in mind that you're probably more aware of any changes in speech than anyone else is. But any time you speak out loud—whether reading or just talking to yourself in the car—you help yourself accommodate more quickly," says Dr. Wiebelt.

Videotape yourself. A videotape can help, suggests Dr. Murrell. A videotape allows you to see what others see when you're talking. And a dentist can use the pictures to determine any problems in jaw or lip movements.

Massage your gums. To relieve sore gums associated with new dentures, massage your gums several times a day, following this routine recommended by Richard Shepard, D.D.S., a dentist in Durango, Colorado. Place your thumb and index finger over your gum, with your index finger on the outside. Massage each section of sore gum by squeezing and rubbing with your thumb and finger. This will promote circulation and give your gums a healthy firmness.

Drink a lot of water. New denture wearers often suffer from either dry mouth or excessive saliva. Either way, frequent sips of water will solve the problem, says Dr. Wiebelt. "Excessive saliva results because the mouth can't tell the difference between the dentures and food in the early going. By sipping water, you wash away the excessive saliva that can cause a gagging or sick feeling." Sucking on hard candy also helps dry mouth, but sipping water is better, especially for people who are overweight, have diabetes or suffer from serious tooth decay.

Don't use adhesives. If you're having trouble with dentures slipping, don't reach for a denture adhesive. If you continually add denture creams and powder, a layer builds up between gums and dentures, which can cause the gum and bone to shrink over time, says Dr. Wiebelt. "The best thing to do is just wait it out, because slipping problems usually end in a week or so. If they last longer, there's probably a problem with the fit, and you should see your dentist." If you *must* use adhesives, be sure to clean your dentures and your gums thoroughly each night to remove all the adhesive.

DIARRHEA

As they say in football, the best offense is a good defense. And diarrhea is your body's best *offensive* defense. Whether its much-ballyhooed revenge can be blamed on Montezuma, the blue plate special, a disagreeable antibiotic, a sneaky viral infection or even stress, diarrhea is the body's painful way of saying "No, thanks!"

Sure, diarrhea lacks a certain something in elegance, but it sure makes up for it in effectiveness. A couple of trips to the toilet (okay, so maybe *more* than just a couple) and you're usually back on your feet. Although it typically takes nature anywhere from two to four days to run this course, here's how to help take the kick out of the "runs."

Be clear on your diet. Most folks know that liquids are the suggested nourishment for the first 24 hours when diarrhea hits. But don't assume that any old liquid will do. "You should take only clear liquids: If you can't see through it, stay away from it," says William B. Ruderman, M.D., chairman of the Department of Gastroenterology at the Cleveland Clinic–Florida in Fort Lauderdale and an expert on diarrhea. "That means you *should* consume soda, tea, bouillon and apple juice. Sports drinks like Gatorade are especially good, because they replace sugars and electrolytes (potassium and sodium). But *avoid* acidic citrus juices, such as orange and grapefruit, and *especially* tomato juice." Exceptions? Beer doesn't qualify, even though you can see through it. Nor do wine, clear alcohol and mixed drinks. In fact, too much beer, wine or any other kind of alcohol can cause diarrhea.

Food-wise, the best choices after the initial 24 hours include "translucent" foods like chicken broth and Jell-O. Whatever you choose to eat at this time should be bland and easily digested.

Make the milk connection. "One of the leading causes of diarrhea in this country is lactose intolerance," says William Y. Chey, M.D., professor of medicine at the University of Rochester School of Medicine and Dentistry in New York.

While few of our experts agree that lactose intolerance is the *leading* cause (most say viral infection), all agree that it is a *major* cause of diarrhea among unsuspecting adults.

"Lactose intolerance can have its onset when you're just a baby, or it can kick in suddenly during your adult years," says Dr. Chey. "You're drinking milk and the next thing you know— bam!—you have gas, pain and diarrhea."

The cure, of course, is to avoid lactose-containing foods, which means staying away from most dairy products, with the exception of yogurt and some aged cheeses, such as cheddar. "Once you do that," says Dr. Chey, "it stops by itself."

Get cultured with yogurt. One of the few exceptions to the clear cuisine rule is yogurt, whose active cultures contain the "good" bacteria your bowel loses to the "bad" bacteria that prompted the diarrhea. "Yogurt is especially effective when the diarrhea is caused by food poisoning," says Manfred Kroger, Ph.D., professor of food science at Pennsylvania State University in University Park. "And it's also effective when diarrhea is the result of stress or antibiotic or radiation treatment. Basically, yogurt's active cultures help Mother Nature speed up the process of replacing the beneficial benign bacteria, and it makes you feel a lot better faster." If yogurt isn't your thing, any acidophilus or fermented dairy product will do. Check the supermarket's dairy case.

Exercise your sweet tooth. A spoonful of sugar helps your body hold on to whatever you're drinking. "Glucose aids the absorption of water by the gut, so if you have sugar in whatever you're taking, you can absorb it more easily," says Dr. Ruderman. "If you're drinking tea or apple juice, add a teaspoonful of sugar to aid in absorption. If you're drinking soda, stick with regular sugared types and stay away from 'diet' varieties." (If you *do* drink soda, he adds, open the cap and let the soda go flat before you imbibe.)

Forget about high fiber—for now. Now's not the time for bran and other high-fiber foods or complex carbohydrates. "It's unwise to stress your system with a lot of nonabsorbable fiber," adds Dr. Ruderman. "When you have diarrhea, the blander, the better." And go for light foods such as cooked carrots, applesauce, baked chicken (without the skin) and other things that don't cause gas. Avoid pasta, corn, oats and most fruits, particularly prunes, pears and apples. Also, have some bananas: Diarrhea can cause potassium depletion, and bananas are high in potassium.

Be anti-antacid. Yesterday's heartburn often becomes today's diarrhea, especially when you treat it with over-the-counter medications. "Antacids are the most common cause of drug-related diarrhea," says Harris Clearfield, M.D., professor of medicine and director of the Division of Gastroenterology at Hahnemann University Hospital in Philadelphia. "Maalox and Mylanta both have magnesium hydroxide in them, which acts exactly like milk of magnesia, making these antacids a common cause of diarrhea." Meanwhile, antacids with aluminum hydroxide, such as Riopan and Amphojel, can cause constipation. (True, this is the opposite effect, but it's just as unwanted.)

Keep drinking. "The more you drink, the better you'll be," says Dr. Ruderman. "Even if you're not thirsty, it's important to take in a lot of fluids, because diarrhea can cause dehydration." His advice? At *least* 6 to 8 ounces every two hours. "You should drink between two and three liters a day," Dr. Ruderman adds. That's the equivalent of 1½ 32-ounce bottles of soda.

Note: Drink even more if you feel thirsty, experience sunken eyeballs or haven't urinated in the past six hours. And drink a lot if your tongue feels very dry or your lips become dry and start to crack.

If you must—take something to stem the tide. Our experts insist that letting diarrhea "run its course" is the best medicine going. If, however, you absolutely must go someplace and be in control of your bodily functions while there, an over-the-counter product called Imodium, available in capsule or liquid form, is probably your best bet for slowing the flow.

"Imodium is very effective," says Dr. Clearfield. "It works by

WHEN DIARRHEA DEMANDS AN M.D.

Diarrhea should usually disappear in one or two days and leave you only slightly worse for wear. In infants, small children, elderly people or those already sick or dehydrated from another illness, however, acute diarrhea can be particularly severe and demands prompt medical attention.

Medical help is also needed if diarrhea does not subside within three or four days, or if it's accompanied by fever and severe abdominal cramps, or if it occurs with rashes, jaundice (yellowing of the skin and whites of the eyes) or extreme weakness. If blood, pus or mucus is found in the stools, call your doctor.

"The most immediate risk associated with acute diarrhea is dehydration," says Harris Clearfield, M.D., professor of medicine and director of the Division of Gastroenterology at Hahnemann University Hospital in Philadelphia. "So if an individual is having a major bout of diarrhea and isn't taking in any food or drink during that time, you're looking at a medical emergency." Seek help, he says.

causing the bowel to tighten up, and by doing so, it prevents things from moving along."

Imodium isn't your only choice. Hydrophilic (*hydro* means water, and *phili* means love) products, such as Kaopectate and Pepto-Bismol, may be useful in the treatment of mild diarrhea.

Don't assume you'll be in the pink with the pink stuff. If you think diarrhea is the result of something you ate and you also have a fever, don't take Pepto-Bismol. The medication slows down "gut motility"—that is, the speed at which the food moves through your system—so the bad stuff stays in your body longer. However, if you have familiar traveler's diarrhea, *without* fever, Pepto-Bismol may help.

DRIVER FATIGUE

Whoever said that "getting there is half the fun" no doubt spent more time coming up with catchy slogans than going places in his car. The fact is, long stretches behind the wheel can be downright boring. And that boredom itself can be dangerous.

"People are more likely to get drowsy and fall asleep when they're in boring and monotonous situations," explains Saul Rothenberg, Ph.D., assistant director of the Sleep Disorder Service and Research Center at Rush–St. Luke's–Presbyterian Medical Center in Chicago. "And driving can be *very* boring and monotonous." No wonder experts believe snoozing behind the wheel is second only to boozing as the leading cause of traffic fatalities.

While the vast majority of long-distance travelers don't fall asleep while driving, many (commuters included) do fall victim to driver fatigue—and fatigue is almost as risky as drowsiness. Symptoms include glazed eyes or a fixed stare, slowed reaction time, forgetfulness, failure to scan the roadway or a tendency to drift toward one side. But there are ways to stay wide-eyed, so you can keep on truckin' safely.

Watch how (and what) you eat. The only thing that will zap your energy and alertness quicker than skipping a meal is eating a big one.

"Driving on a full stomach is not a good idea because of post-meal sleepiness," says Dr. Rothenberg. "In order to maintain driver alertness, it's better to eat lightly."

Low-fat protein may be the best choice to avoid drowsiness, some experts say. Good sources of low-fat protein include lean meats, poultry, fish, yogurt and low-fat cottage cheese. Carbohydrates to avoid include potatoes, corn, bagels, muffins and *especially* snack foods like chips and crackers.

Keep your car's interior cool. "A warm car can enhance sleepiness, so try to keep your car as cool as possible," says Dr.

Rothenberg. "Cold invigorates—especially when you're tired—so open a window or turn on the air-conditioning."

Snooze the night before. Many people get driver fatigue on long-distance trips because they simply didn't get enough sleep the night before. They were too busy with packing and other pre-departure hassles.

"If you know you'll be putting in long hours driving, the easiest thing to do is go to bed an hour or two earlier than normal, so you can get a better-than-usual night's sleep," says Timothy Roehrs, Ph.D., director of research at the Henry Ford Hospital Sleep Disorders and Research Center in Detroit.

Adjust your body clock—before you leave. Even more effective for long trips is to adjust your body clock so that you'll be alert during times you normally get drowsy.

For instance, if you want to do late-night driving, start going to bed one hour later each night (and rising one hour later) for three or four consecutive nights, starting about one week before departure, advises Maria Simonson, Ph.D., Sc.D., professor emeritus and director of the Health, Weight and Stress Program at Johns Hopkins Medical Institutions in Baltimore. If you want to hit the road before the rooster crows, hit the sack an hour earlier every night during the week before you leave.

If all else fails, pull over. "If you find yourself losing your edge, pull off in a safe place and take a 20- to 30-minute nap," says Deborah Freund, a transportation specialist with the Federal Highway Administration in Washington, D.C., and project manager of a long-term study on driver fatigue. Be sure that you give yourself enough time to wake up fully before you start to drive again.

DRY HAIR

The average human head has 150,000 hairs, and, conformists that they are, when one's dry, they're all dry. But unlike a dry flower garden or polished rice, the solution is not simply to add water. Water, in fact, may be responsible for the hair's parched condition, particularly if we're talking about water of the salty, chlorinated or sudsy variety.

Swimming and overshampooing are two common causes of arid, fly-away locks, says Jack Myers, director of the National Cosmetology Association. Other culprits, he says, can include colorings, permanents, electric curlers, excessive blow-dry and too much exposure to wind and sun.

Here's a quick course on how to rescue dried-out hair.

Shampoo with care. "It's in vogue these days to shampoo every day, but shampooing doesn't only wash away dirt, it washes out the hair's protective oils," says Thomas Goodman, Jr., M.D., a dermatologist and assistant professor at the University of Tennessee Center for Health Sciences in Memphis. If you've dried your hair out from too much lather, give your hair a needed break—try washing less often. And use only a mild shampoo, one labeled "for dry or damaged hair."

Use a conditioner. When hair becomes dry, the outer layers, called cuticles, peel off from the central shaft. Conditioners glue the cuticles back to the shaft, add lubricant to the hair and prevent static electricity (which creates frizz). Pick a conditioner that works well for you and use it after every shampoo, says Dr. Goodman.

Don't hold the mayo. "Mayonnaise makes an excellent conditioner," says David Daines, owner of David Daines Salon in New York City. He advises a regular mayo bath—once a week or so. Put a dollop in the palm of your hand, then work it into your hair for *at least* five minutes before washing it out. (The preferred time for a full-blown mayo treatment is an hour, according to Daines.)

Spray on the brew. If mayo is a little too messy for your taste, you can still get help from the flip-top section of your refrigerator. "Beer is a wonderful setting lotion that gives a crisp, healthy, shiny look—even to dry hair," says Daines. Pour some of the brew into an empty pump-bottle. Then spray it onto your hair *after* you've shampooed and towel-dried but *before* you blow-dry or style. And don't worry about smelling like a lush—the odor of the beer quickly disperses.

Don't swim bareheaded. "Chlorine is one of the most destructive things to hair," says Steven Docherty, senior art director at New York City's Vidal Sassoon Salon. So make a rubber cap part of your regular swim attire. For extra protection, he says, first rub a little olive oil into your hair.

Dry without heat. Two of the most intense sources of heat—and damage—are curling irons and electric curlers, says Joanne Harris, who operates the Joanne Harris Salon in Los Angeles and whose clients include many Hollywood stars. She suggests you rediscover the unheated plastic cylinder rollers that were used in years gone by.

For straightening, wrap slightly moist hair under and around the cold rollers, as if you were creating a pageboy hairdo. Leave them in place for about ten minutes. For curling or adding wave, try using sponge rollers overnight or sleeping with moist braids. Since blow-drying is also damaging, gently pat hair dry with a towel.

Wear a hat. One of the easiest ways to avoid dry hair is simply to wear a hat during windy weather. "Whipping winds can fray your hair like a piece of fabric," says Michael Ramsey, M.D., clinical instructor of dermatology at Baylor College of Medicine in Houston. Plus, a hat helps protect hair from the sun, which can also dry hair.

Snip off split ends. What to do about split ends? Snip 'em off, suggests Dr. Goodman. One round of quick snips every six weeks or so should keep those frayed ends under control.

DRY MOUTH

Ever notice how drooling seems to come naturally to the very young? From the mouths of innocent babes comes enough saliva to turn a bib to a bath mat. But as we grow up, we tend to dry up. The addition of years seems to translate to a loss of saliva.

Aging alone, however, isn't the only cause of xerostomia, or dry mouth. More often we can blame it on all the 24-carat hassles that we live with in the golden age of our lives: Most cases of dry mouth can be blamed on some 400 medicines used to treat nearly everything from arthritis to ulcers. Even caffeine and over-the-counter pain relievers such as ibuprofen can contribute to dry mouth.

Besides making your mouth feel like it's plugged with cotton, dry mouth can make swallowing, eating and even talking difficult. Worst case: Mouth tissue becomes cracked and irritated, and you begin to suffer related problems such as bad breath, lost fillings, gum infections and tooth decay. But here's how to permanently wet your whistle if you're among the one in three Americans with dry mouth.

Take a hard line against soft drinks. Drinking more is the obvious solution to dry mouth—as long as you're not slurping soda, orange juice or other beverages that contain either citric or phosphoric acid. "Soft drinks are very acidic, and people with dry mouth lack the saliva necessary to neutralize these acids that can harm the teeth," says James Sciubba, D.M.D., Ph.D., chairman of the Department of Dental Medicine at Long Island Jewish Medical Center in New Hyde Park, New York, and founding chairman of the Sjögren's Syndrome Foundation. Instead, carrying a flask of water and taking frequent sips is the best way to get your mouth moist again. "The key is how frequently you drink, not necessarily how much you drink," he says.

Suck on fruit pits. Pits from peaches, nectarines and cherries help increase saliva flow without adding any calories. Just be careful not to swallow them.

Eat mushy foods. Eating any food will stimulate saliva. But the best choices are soft foods and those moistened with sauces or gravies that go down the hatch easily, says Nelson Rhodus, D.M.D., associate professor of oral medicine at the University of Minnesota in Minneapolis.

Go sugarless. "Use of sugar by a patient with a dry mouth will produce tooth decay within six months," warns Dr. Sciubba. "One of the best ways to keep saliva flowing is to suck on hard candies or to chew gum, but the gum and candy must be sugarless." In fact, sucking on sorbitol-containing sugarless candies, mints and gum has been found to increase saliva tenfold in some people.

Rinse your mouth with some fluoride. When saliva production is low, your risk of cavities and gum disease is high. Swishing with a fluoride mouth rinse at bedtime helps remineralize teeth and can help protect you against cavities and gum disease.

There are also artificial saliva products that help. "In our studies, we found that over-the-counter products such as MouthKote provide a nice, moist coating over mucous membranes," says Dr. Rhodus. Other products include Xero-Lube, Salivart and Evian mineral water spray.

Moisturize the air. Using a cool-air vaporizer in your home is a good way to add much-needed extra humidity to the air—especially if you're a mouth breather, says Dr. Sciubba. But make an effort to *always* breathe through your nose to prevent saliva from evaporating.

Use lemon sparingly. While full-fledged lemonade should be avoided, tasting some lemon juice diluted in water or rinsing with a bit of lemon juice and glycerin is a good way to stimulate the flow of saliva, says Dr. Rhodus. But here's the drawback: If your mucous membranes are so dry that you have developed sores, the citric acid could further irritate your mouth. (If you do have these sores, go light on lemon as well as spicy foods and anything else that can irritate your mouth.)

DRY SKIN AND WINTER ITCH

As winter approaches, our bodies turn toward flannel, our attention turns toward cheap Florida airfares and our skin takes a turn toward something resembling Melba toast.

You can blame that toasted skin on the warm, toasty air that heats our homes, schools and offices. When it gets cold, we naturally warm up the house. The problem is, unless you add humidity to your surroundings with a humidifier or pans of water near radiators, a heated room has only about 15 percent relative humidity—as dry as Death Valley. And that turns our skin dry, flaky, scaly and usually itchy (and *always* bothersome).

Plus, there are other irritants to make matters worse—wind, cold, soaps, water (which dries skin when it evaporates), even added stress. Put it all together and your epidermis can dry out quicker than Aunt Gizelda's holiday fruitcake.

Dry skin and winter itch share a lot of symptoms with eczema and dermatitis, and some of the remedies for those problems can bring relief. But the key to making the winter season a merry one, itch-wise, is keeping your birthday suit well protected. Here's how.

Keep skin moisturized. Probably the most important thing you can do to prevent and treat dry skin is to moisturize *daily* with a cream-based moisturizer, advises Sheryl Clark, M.D., a dermatologist at The New York Hospital–Cornell Medical Center in New York City. "An oil-free moisturizer is recommended for those who tend to break out. Also, those with sensitive skin should choose a moisturizer without perfumes or lanolin." The brands most highly recommended by experts include Eucerin, Complex-15, Moisturel, Aquaphor and Aquaderm—all available over the counter.

But don't get soaked. You don't need expensive skin creams to keep skin moisturized. "Nothing beats plain petroleum jelly or mineral oil as a moisturizer," says Howard Donsky, M.D., associate professor of medicine at the University of Toronto and author of *Beauty Is Skin Deep*. In fact, he adds, virtually *any* vegetable oil or hyrogenated cooking oil—from Crisco Oil to sunflower or peanut oil—can be used to relieve dry skin. But note: They do feel greasier than commercial moisturizers.

Don't be too hyper about your hygiene. "Bathe in cool to tepid water as briefly as possible and no more than once a day," advises Michael Ramsey, M.D., clinical instructor of dermatology at Baylor College of Medicine in Houston. "Cleansing lotions are more gentle than soaps, and they're just as effective at removing dirt," adds Leonard Swinyer, M.D., clinical professor of medicine at the University of Utah in Salt Lake City. And *don't* use a washcloth—just your fingertips. If you must use soaps, stick with mild brands such as Dove, Aveeno or Basis.

Select superfatted soaps. "Most soaps have lye in them," says Hillard H. Pearlstein, M.D., assistant clinical professor of dermatology at the Mount Sinai School of Medicine in New York City, "and while lye is great for cleaning, it's very irritating to dry skin." He recommends that people with dry skin avoid strong soaps such as Dial or Ivory and reach instead for "superfatted" soaps like Basis, Neutrogena or Dove. Superfatted soaps have extra amounts of fatty substances—cold cream, cocoa butter, coconut oil or lanolin—added during the manufacturing process.

"A product like Dove, for instance, isn't really a soap at all," Dr. Pearlstein says. "It's more like a cold cream." But such are the trade-offs in the skin game. Though they don't clean as well, "the superfatted soaps are less irritating to dry skin," he says, "and they do make a difference."

Add some oil to your bath. Make the most of your tub time by adding a bath oil rich in moisturizers—even when you apply creams *after* bathing. Again, there's no need for the fancy stuff: Plain ol' castor oil is an excellent, low-cost choice. "It's one of the few oils that will disperse in water, and it won't leave a ring around the tub," says Varro E. Tyler, Ph.D., professor of pharmacognosy at Purdue University in West Lafayette, Indiana, and author of *The Honest Herbal.*

Make your own bath oil by mixing ½ cup of castor oil with ten drops of sandlewood-, pine-, rosemary- or mint-scented oil and storing it in a closed jar. Add one teaspoon of the mixture each time you bathe. For those who prefer store-bought brands, Alpha Keri body oil, Geri-Bath and Nutraderm bath oil are highly recommended. *Caution:* Be careful in the bathroom, because these oils can make tubs and floors extremely slippery.

Dry yourself damp. After bathing, pat your skin almost dry—never totally dry—with a towel. While the skin is still damp, apply your moisturizing lotion. "It's more effective to apply moisturizer to damp skin *immediately* after bathing than to put it on totally dry skin, because the moisturizer is what holds the water in," says Kenneth H. Neldner, M.D., professor and chairman of the Department of Dermatology at Texas Tech University Health Sciences Center in Lubbock. "A couple of pats with a towel will make you as dry as you want to be before you apply the lotion. You're trying to trap a little water in the skin, and that's the fundamental rule in fighting off dryness." If you have dry hands, he advises keeping some moisturizer near each sink in the house and using it as needed.

Keep it cool. One good way to combat winter itch is as easy as reaching for your thermostat and turning it down. "Keeping your house on the cool side in the winter might help," says Dr. Pearlstein. "That's because cool air has an anesthetic effect—it makes your skin feel good." When you heat your house too much, he explains, it makes blood vessels dilate, and when blood vessels dilate, the itch/tingle cycle begins. "But when you cool skin, either by cool water or cool air, it feels good," Dr. Pearlstein says. "And skin tends to be less itchy if you keep it on the cool side."

Be wary of wool. Clothing made of wool—or any other fuzzy or heavy material—can be particularly irritating to excessively dry skin, says Stephen M. Purcell, D.O., chairman of the Department of Dermatology at Philadelphia College of Osteopathic Medicine and assistant clinical professor at Hahnemann University School of Health Sciences in Philadelphia. "The last thing itchy skin needs is to have something scratchy over it. Cotton is probably the best material to wear, since polyester blends can also be irritating to some people."

Shave *before* bedtime. Shaving is tough enough on your tender skin, but meeting the cold reality of Old Man Winter right afterward makes your dry skin even worse, adds Dr. Swinyer. Unless you're hampered by severe five o'clock shadow, shave before bedtime, when your puss won't be subjected to such a drastic change in temperature.

And avoid eye-opening after-shaves. Their high alcohol content is too drying and zaps remaining moisture during this mean season, adds Dr. Swinyer.

Wear baggy, loose-fitting clothing. Besides being more abrasive, tighter clothing traps perspiration, which softens the outer layer of skin, breaks down its protective barrier and worsens dry skin, says dermatologist Rodney Basler, M.D., assistant professor of internal medicine at the University of Nebraska Medical Center in Omaha. But looser-fitting clothes, particularly in "breathable" fabrics like cotton, allow perspiration to be absorbed naturally.

EARWAX BUILDUP

Earwax is a recycling center. Most of the time, your ears produce just enough protective wax to trap dust in your ear canal and move it to the ear opening. Then the wax and dust are bathed away whenever you wash around your ears.

But sometimes the wax gets all jammed up—which is uncomfortable, annoying and sometimes downright itchy. Not only that, wax-plugged ears are more susceptible to infection. So if you find yourself with too much wax, here's how to deal with it.

Irrigate earwax. "Gently irrigate your ear with body-temperature water," suggests Stephen P. Cass, M.D., assistant professor of otolaryngology at the Eye and Ear Institute of Pittsburgh.

To do it right, you'll need a rubber ear syringe (available at most pharmacies) and a sinkful of water. (If it's the correct temperature, it will feel neither warm nor cold when you dip your hand in.) Hold your head over the sink while you very gently squirt the water into your ear, letting water and wax run out into the sink. Be sure to dry the ear canal after washing. To do this, fill an eyedropper with rubbing alcohol and squeeze the alcohol into the ear. It will absorb moisture and dry the ear.

If you're prone to excess buildup of wax, use the syringe to irrigate your ears this way once or twice a month as a precaution, suggests Jerome C. Goldstein, M.D., executive vice president of the American Academy of Otolaryngology and Head and Neck Surgery in Alexandria, Virginia. (But you shouldn't squirt anything in your ear if you have any kind of eardrum damage—so check with your doctor first, and again if you feel any pain.)

Baby your ears. If the wax refuses to budge, you may need to soften it up before you irrigate. One way is to use baby oil, according to Anthony J. Yonkers, M.D., chairman of the Department of Otolaryngology and Head and Neck Surgery at the University of Nebraska Medical Center in Omaha. "Warm up the oil to body temperature, then place a few drops into the ear twice a

DO YOU HAVE TOO LITTLE OF A GOOD THING?

Yes, it is possible to have too *little* earwax. People who have skin conditions like eczema and psoriasis some-times have an earwax deficit.

The cure?

"People can replenish earwax by putting a coat of Vaseline in the ear canal," says Anthony J. Yonkers, M.D., chairman of the Department of Otolaryngology and Head and Neck Surgery at the University of Nebraska Medical Center in Omaha. Use your finger to apply the coating to the outer edges of the ear opening only.

And if your wax shortage causes itching, augment this treat-ment with an over-the-counter itch reliever such as hydrocorti-sone cream, suggests Stephen P. Cass, M.D., assistant professor of otolaryngology at the Eye and Ear Institute of Pittsburgh. Apply the cream to the outer ear, and the itching should ease in a few days.

day. It will melt or soften the wax, and you can irrigate it out," Dr. Yonkers says.

Try peroxide. Another softening-up method: "Fill the ear with a dropperful of peroxide, and let it bubble and work for five minutes or so," suggests Dr. Goldstein. If you need to, put a piece of cotton in the opening of the ear canal, so you can sit up while the peroxide goes to work. Then flush it away with water.

Clear your canals with nonprescription treatments. Many over-the-counter earwax treatments, such as Murine and Debrox, are actually lubricant-based peroxide solutions. "They work, too," says Frank Marlowe, M.D., an otolaryngologist for the Medical College of Pennsylvania in Philadelphia. Plus you get a side benefit from the lubricant: It relieves dry skin in the ear canal. (That dry skin can become enmeshed with wax, causing formation of a wax ball that blocks the ear canal.)

A stool softener might sit well with you. If you have impacted wax, try using Colace, a stool softener found in most drugstores, suggests Dr. Cass. Using an eyedropper, put a couple of drops of liquid Colace in each ear. You can leave it there from a few minutes to an hour or two (depending on how stubborn the wax is), then irrigate your ears with water.

Don't use a Pik or a poke. No matter how much earwax accumulates in your ears, don't be tempted to probe for it with paper clips, tweezers or any small object—*including cotton-tipped swabs*—warns Dr. Cass. You'll push wax farther into your ear, and you might scratch or damage an eardrum. And don't use a Water Pik–type device—that's for teeth only. If you're going to irrigate your ears, use *only* an ear syringe.

Blow-dry your ears. Don't rub your ears dry, say doctors. Instead, dry your ears with a hair dryer. Do this after the irrigating procedure and also every time you shower.

EYESTRAIN

Eyestrain can happen to anyone. In fact, it usually happens to *everyone,* especially if you're over age 40. You're likely to have eyestrain at least occasionally if you use a computer, watch TV, drive a car or live in a smoggy city.

You know you've got eyestrain when normally clear images (such as words on the computer screen or print on the page) begin to appear blurry. Your eyes start to ache so much that you just want to close them for a while. Well, that's one thing you can do. But here are some other ways you can put a lid on eyestrain.

Take a tea break. Warm eyebright tea is a gentle balm for eyes that are strained. "Take a towel and soak it in brewed eyebright tea," says Meir Schneider, director of the Center for Self Healing in San Francisco and author of *Self Healing: My Life and Vision.* "Lie down, place the warm towel over your closed eyes and leave it there for 10 to 15 minutes. It will make your eyestrain go away."

Be very careful not to let the towel drip tea into your eyes, though—and be sure the tea has cooled down enough before you soak the towel in it. *Note:* Eyebright tea is not a real tea but a mixture of herbal ingredients, sold in loose tea form at most health food stores, specifically for eyestrain.

Take time-outs from close work. "When you're using a computer or doing any other type of close work that strains your eyes, stop every hour for about two minutes and give your eyes a rest," suggests Eric Donnenfeld, M.D., associate professor of ophthalmology at North Shore University Hospital–Cornell Medical College in Manhasset, New York. Just close your eyes and do nothing for a couple of minutes."

Stop reading—and refocus. "When you're reading, stop every 30 minutes or so and focus on something far away for a few seconds," adds Merrill M. Knopf, M.D., an ophthalmologist in Long Beach, California, and an officer of the California Association of Ophthalmology. There's a muscle in your eye that contracts when you're doing close-up work, Dr. Knopf explains. By refocusing, you relieve the spasms in that eye muscle. If you want something to look at, hang a sheet of newspaper on a far wall and try to read the larger print.

Put your eyes "on the blink." Your eyes have their own personal masseuse—the eyelids. "Make it a point to consciously blink your eyes frequently and not squint," says Schneider. "Each blink cleanses your eyes and gives them a tiny little massage."

Exercise your eyes. Standing about five feet from a blank wall, have someone toss a tennis ball at the wall while you try to catch it each time it bounces off. Or hold your thumb out at arm's length. Move it in circles and Xs, bringing the thumb closer, then farther away, as you follow it with your eyes. Both exercises help offset damage caused by eyestrain and improve the brain-to-nerve-to-muscle connection of your vision, says Don Teig, O.D., an optometrist and sports vision specialist in Ridgefield, Connecticut.

Pay attention to lighting. "It doesn't hurt your eyes to read in dim light, but you can strain them if the light doesn't provide enough contrast," says Samuel L. Guillory, M.D., a New York City ophthalmologist and assistant clinical professor at Mount Sinai Medical Center of the City University of New York. "Use a soft light that gives contrast, but not glare, when you read. And don't use any lamp that reflects light directly back into your eyes."

Darken your screen. Those aren't just letters and numbers on your screen. They're also tiny light bulbs that send light directly into your eyes. You need to turn the wattage down, so to speak. "Don't make the letters too bright," advises Dr. Guillory. "Turn the brightness down to a dim level and then adjust the contrast to make up the difference." An added tip: Take a pencil and make a mark on the knob you adjusted. Then make a corresponding mark on the computer. That way you'll just have to realign the marks if somebody changes the setting on your computer.

FATIGUE

Be honest. When you first heard the words "energy crisis," did you think of Arab oil embargoes or yourself? Everyone, at one time or another, feels fatigued. And who wouldn't like to have more energy than they now have?

Unfortunately, having more energy is a lot like having more money— it's easier to talk about it than to get it. Yet it's also easier to increase your energy than you probably realize. Of course, the broad prescription from doctors is still the same: Get plenty of rest, eat a balanced diet and exercise. But here physicians and other authorities on fatigue go beyond these generalities and offer more specific, high-octane suggestions.

So, ladies and gentlemen, please start your engines.

Eat a three-piece breakfast. The three components of a good breakfast are carbohydrates, proteins and fats, advises Rick Ricer, M.D., assistant professor of clinical family medicine at Ohio State University College of Medicine in Columbus. Of course you don't want to *add* fat to your breakfast table. You will get plenty of fats, a good form of storable energy, in the proteins you eat.

But even cereal (a complex carbohydrate) with milk (a source of protein) can get your day off to a good start. Wheat toast and muffins are also good complex carbohydrate options. For protein, you might want to consider low-fat yogurt and cottage cheese, or a small piece of chicken or fish.

Meanwhile, Dr. Ricer warns not to eat an ultra-high carbohydrate breakfast laden with simple sugars. "You can actually overactivate your insulin and your blood sugar will drop: that can leave you jittery." So avoid the doughnut shop between home and office.

Work out to rev up. "Exercise actually gives you energy," says Vicky Young, M.D., an assistant professor in the Department of Preventive Medicine at the Medical College of Wisconsin in Milwaukee. Study after study supports those words, including one by the National Aeronautics and Space Administration. More than 200 federal employees were placed on a moderate, regular exercise program. The results: 90 percent said they had never felt better. Almost half said they felt less stress, and almost one-third reported they slept better.

Dr. Young recommends giving yourself a dose of energetic exercise— brisk walking is enough—three to five times a week, for 20 to 30 minutes each time and no later than 2 hours before bedtime.

Tackle one thing at a time. "Make lists," says David Sheridan, M.D., an associate professor in the Department of Preventive Medicine at the University of South Carolina School of Medicine in Columbia. "Many times, people feel fatigued because they think, 'I have so much to do I don't know where to start.'" By setting priorities and charting your progress as you make your way through the list, you can remain focused and energetic.

Take one a day. If you are guilty of missing meals, dieting or not eating properly, Dr. Young says, taking one multivitamin and mineral supplement a day is a good idea. "A lack of good nutrition can cause fatigue, and a supplement can help make up for the missing nutrients. But don't look to a vitamin to give you instant energy," says Dr. Ricer.

"It's a fallacy that when you're tired you just take more vitamins and feel better" Dr. Ricer says. Only eating properly can do that.

Add some stress to your life. It's no surprise that too much stress can knock you out. But if there's not *enough* stress in your life, you can feel fatigued because of boredom and lack of motivation. "It's sort of like the tension or stress on a violin string," says Paul J. Rosch, M.D., clinical professor of medicine and psychiatry at New York Medical College in Vallhalla and president of the American Institute of Stress in Yonkers. "If you have too much, the string will snap. If you have too little, you'll get a dull, raspy sound. But just the right amount creates a beautiful tone. Similarly, we need to find the right amount of stress that allows us to make beautiful music in our lives."

The key is to add the kind of stress that will make you feel challenged, not beaten. "I suggest becoming a volunteer," says consumer health expert John Renner, M.D., clinical professor of family medicine at the University of Missouri at Kansas City. The only additional stress is your commitment to show up on time and do the job, but you have the challenge of working with people and producing results.

But avoid stress carriers. "Some people are Typhoid Marys of stress, and just being around them can fatigue you," says Maria Simonson, Ph.D., Sc.D., professor emeritus and director of the Health, Weight and Stress Program at Johns Hopkins Medical Institutions in Baltimore. "They tend to be the people who are insensitive, complainers and blamers. The best thing you can do is try to stay clear of them."

Color your world. "If you live in a dark, dark house, you're going to feel fatigued," says Dr. Ricer. Add some color and more light to your life, he suggests. Studies show that wearing red or being in red surroundings energizes. The color green has been found to evoke peacefulness and serenity, while brown helps induce feelings of warmness and camaraderie.

Lose weight . . . but not too quickly. It's true, lugging around extra weight can tire you out faster, but don't try to lose too much too soon. Crash diets can send your energy into a nosedive. (Because ultra-low-calorie diets concentrate on one type of food, such as grapefruit, they don't give you all the nutrients you need for sufficient energy.)

When your calorie intake is restricted too much, it's very stressful for the body, according to Manfred Kroger, Ph.D., professor of food science at Pennsylvania State University in University Park. "And one of the many symptoms of this type of stress is fatigue."

For responsible dieting, men should consume at least 1,500 calories a day, and women should have 1,200 calories or more.

OPEN YOUR MIND TO ENERGY

Where your mind goes, your body goes. That the mind can influence the body is now generally accepted. But have you accepted it? Are you aware that your thoughts can have a lot to do with how tired you feel?

Well, they can. So here are some beneficial attitudes that can affect your energy level.

- Think positive. Championship athletes do it, successful corporate executive officers do it and you should do it.
- Be motivated. When you think about it, it's pretty hard to do much of anything if you're not motivated. But it's next to impossible to accomplish tasks that require mega-energy if your spirit just isn't in it.
- Be confident. Chances are good that if you feel you can do it, you will have the energy to do it. And once you've proven to yourself that you've got the energy, you will become even more confident.

Turn off the tube. Sure, television helps you unwind after a hard day of hassles—but maybe you're unwinding too much. TV is notorious for lulling folks into a state of lethargy. Instead of watching the tube, try something a little more mentally stimulating, like reading, says Dr. Ricer. "That will be more energizing."

Put out the fire. Doctors always advise giving up smoking, but add this to the list of reasons: Smoking adversely affects the delivery of oxygen to tissues. The result is fatigue.

When you first quit, however, don't expect an immediate energy boost. Nicotine acts as a stimulant, and withdrawal may cause some temporary tiredness.

FLATULENCE

I t's tough to be serious about flatulence, though we promise to try. It's tough because even the scientists who study the subject poke fun at their own research, writing of failed experiments that ended "without even a whiff of success."

Yes, the pun was intended and was in very bad taste, but such is the nature of this science—even at the highest levels. Consider Michael D. Levitt, M.D., one of the top researchers in the field. His peers know him as "the man who brought status to flatus and class to gas." In his own words, Dr. Levitt describes his work as "an attempt to pump some data into a field filled largely with hot air."

Hot air, perhaps, and a colorful history as well. Hippocrates investigated flatulence extensively, and ancient physicians who specialized in it became known as "pneumatists." In early American history, such great men as Benjamin Franklin taxed their minds seeking a cure for "escaped wind."

In more recent times, Stephen Goldfinger, M.D., a digestive disease expert, wrote that "glaring at the next guy, when all else fails, can make life easier." Yes, it's tough to be serious about flatulence, but we promise to try. Read on.

Lay off the lactose. "If you are lactose intolerant, you could have flatulence problems from eating dairy foods," says Dennis Savaiano, Ph.D., associate professor of food science and nutrition at the University of Minnesota in Minneapolis. Lactose-intolerant people have a low intestinal level of the enzyme lactase, which is needed to digest lactose, the type of sugar found in many dairy foods.

But you don't necessarily need to be diagnosed as lactose intolerant to have unwanted repercussions. Some people can handle only certain amounts and different kinds of milk products with comfort. If you or your doctor suspects that your favorite dairy product is causing your problem, try eating it in smaller servings or along with a meal for a day or two until you notice where gas begins to be a problem.

Take time for tea. Peppermint, spearmint, anise and caraway contain oils that settle the stomach, acording to William J. Keller, Ph.D., professor and head of the Division of Medicinal Chemistry and Pharmaceutics at Northeast Louisiana University School of Pharmacy in Monroe and secretary of the American Society of Pharmacognosy. "Herbal tea is a good form to take them in," he says. And they taste good. Spearmint and peppermint teas are readily available in the tea section of your supermarket; anise and caraway may require a stop at the health food store.

Avoid gas-promoting foods. The primary cause of flatulence is the digestive system's inability to absorb certain carbohydrates, says Samuel Klein, M.D., assistant professor of gastroenterology and human nutrition at the University of Texas Medical School at Galveston.

Though you probably know that beans are sure-fire flatus producers, many people don't realize that cabbage, broccoli, brussels sprouts, onions, cauliflower, whole wheat flour, radishes, bananas, apricots, pretzels and many more foods can also be highly flatugenic.

Get quick relief with popular OTCs. While many physicians are recommending activated charcoal for relief of intestinal gas, pharmacists say simethicone-containing products are still the most popular with consumers. Among the over-the-counter favorites: Gas-X, Maalox Plus, Mylanta II and Mylicon.

Unlike activated charcoal's absorbent action, simethicone's defoaming action relieves flatulence by dispersing and preventing the formation of mucous-surrounded gas pockets in the stomach and intestines.

Remember the two Ps. Think posture and position. If you have a problem with gas, you should probably be eating your meals when you're sitting at the table, not when you're lounging or lying down. "When you drink or eat lying down, the gas in your stomach cannot escape," says W. Steven Pray, Ph.D., R.Ph., professor in the Southwestern Oklahoma State University School

BEAN CUISINE: GETTING THE GAS OUT

I f you love beans and legumes but hate living with the consequences, there is a solution.

Clearly, beans and legumes cause flatulence, although the better they're cooked, the less the problem. Indeed, beans seem to lose a lot of their gas-producing properties in water. Studies have shown that soaking beans for 12 hours or germinating them on damp paper towels for 24 hours can significantly reduce the amount of gas-producing compounds. In fact, soaking followed by 30 minutes of pressure cooking at 15 pounds per square inch reduced the compounds by up to 90 percent in one study.

of Pharmacy in Weatherford. Slouching can cause problems, too, so watch that posture.

Breathe air, don't swallow it. "Eat slowly, chew thoroughly and don't gulp," says Bruce Yaffe, M.D., a gastroenterologist affiliated with Lenox Hill Hospital in New York City. The reason? "When you gulp, you swallow air, and swallowing air will only make things worse." Chewing gum, ill-fitting dentures and sucking on hard candy can also cause you to swallow a lot of excess air, he says. To avoid those gulps that go to gas, steer clear of carbonated beverages and beer. And it's another reason not to smoke.

Dry up that drip. "The most important thing I've discovered in my medical career," reports Dr. Yaffe, "is that postnasal drip often leads to air swallowing and increased gas production. People who have mucus in the backs of their throats are always swallowing."

FOOT ODOR

What gives? You already wash your feet regularly (with warm soapy water). You change your socks at least once a day. And your shoes are clean enough to prevent high school biology classes from making field trips in your closet to collect mold spore samples.

Still, those dogs of yours smell bad enough to make those around want to howl at the moon in agony. So the next time you remove your shoes (that is, *after* you and the rest of your ZIP code come back to consciousness), try these breath-of-fresh-air remedies for the all-too-common problem of smelly feet.

Take tea and see. "Using a soak made from tea bags eliminates the odor from smelly feet because the tannic acid in the tea literally tans the hide," says Jerome Z. Litt, M.D., assistant clinical professor of dermatology at Case Western Reserve University School of Medicine in Cleveland. "You take a couple of tea bags and boil them in a pint of water for 15 minutes. Then remove the tea bags and pour the pint of strong, hot tea into a basin or a large pot filled with two quarts of cool water. Soak for 30 minutes daily for a week or ten days and you'll have no smelly, sweaty feet."

Heed sage advice. Europeans sometimes sprinkle the fragrant herb sage into their shoes to control odor, says Suzanne M. Levine, D.P.M., clinical assistant podiatrist at Mount Sinai Hospital in New York City. Perhaps a dash of these dry, crumbled leaves will do the trick for you.

Try inserts. Some shoe inserts, such as Johnson's Odor-Eaters, contain activated charcoal, which absorbs moisture and helps control odor. Dr. Levine says these products have helped some of her patients.

Try an acne fighter. "If your feet are really smelly—what I call toxic sock syndrome—examine the bottoms," says Rodney Basler, M.D., a dermatologist and assistant professor of internal

DO YOUR FEET WORK HARDER THAN YOU DO?

Believe it or not, says Bethlehem, Pennsylvania, podiatrist Neal Kramer, D.P.M., sometimes feet perspire a lot because they simply *work* harder than they should. A structural defect (such as flat feet) or a job that keeps you hopping all day could be the underlying culprit. Either would increase the activity of your foot muscles. And the harder your feet work, the more they perspire in an attempt to cool themselves.

Although feet that perspire don't necessarily smell bad, the wetness is an open invitation for bacteria that do produce odor.

"If you correct the underlying problem with an arch support or some other orthotic shoe insert," says Dr. Kramer, "you can actually cut down on the amount of sweat produced. If the muscles don't have to work as hard, they just don't give off as much heat."

medicine at the University of Nebraska Medical Center in Omaha. "If you have whitish soles with tiny pits, then you probably have a condition called pitted keratolysis. And since the organism that brings on this condition is the same species that causes acne, you can get relief by using an over-the-counter acne medication with 10 percent benzoyl peroxide, such as Oxy-10."

Use an antiperspirant. You can buy special foot deodorants, but here's a lower-cost alternative: Use an underarm *antiperspirant*, which controls odor and wetness, says Stephen Weinberg, D.P.M., a podiatrist who specializes in sports medicine at Columbus Hospital in Chicago. (Deodorants, meanwhile, only control odor.) His advice: Use a roll-on that contains the active ingredient aluminum chloride hexahydrate at least twice daily. Aerosols aren't as effective, since a lot of their oomph is lost in the air.

FORGETFULNESS

Hmmmm, now what were we going to discuss next? Oh, yeah, how to cure those blasted bouts of forgetfulness. You know, when a name or date is on the tip of your tongue . . . or you can't seem to remember where you parked your car . . . or left your keys.

Frustrating as it is, a memory slip is hardly uncommon. Everyone has occasional episodes of forgetfulness, so even if you've forgotten the last time it happened to you, here's how to build a better memory.

Get in shape. Scientific research confirms that a healthy body indeed helps breed a healthy mind—memory-wise, at least. Several studies show that people over age 40 who exercise aerobically at least three times a week have 20 percent better memory skills than people who don't exercise.

"Regular exercise improves blood flow to the brain," explains Richard Gordin, Ph.D., professor of physical education at Utah State University in Logan. "And improved blood flow often means improved thinking and memory."

Tune in talk shows. "The most troublesome tasks for everyone are remembering names and faces and remembering dates and appointments. I recommend you watch TV shows that will help improve those skills," says Douglas Herrmann, Ph.D., a research scientist at the National Center for Health Statistics in Hyattsville, Maryland, and author of *Super Memory*. "Since meeting new people challenges memory, watch talk and game shows, and try to recall each guest's name as the show goes on. A show like 'Wheel of Fortune' is good for improving your vocabulary and recalling word definitions."

Write it down. Putting information in writing also puts it into your memory, says Dr. Herrmann. So try writing down important information in order to remember it more easily later on. Many memory experts suggest you "make lists."

KEEP THESE SYMPTOMS IN MIND

Most skin lumps are not cancer, and most slips of memory are not Alzheimer's disease. "But people tend to be hard on themselves, particularly so as they get older," says Stanley Berent, Ph.D.

When is your forgetfulness so serious that you should see a professional about it? Dr. Berent suggests the following guidelines:

- Do you lose contact with reality? It's one thing to forget today's date, another to forget the year. If you lose track of where you are, can't remember if it's evening or morning, or have forgotten the name of your spouse (as opposed to someone you just met), a doctor should be consulted.
- Are you uncomfortable with yourself? If you're feeling anxious about your recent memory lapses, don't sweat it out—seek a doctor's advice.
- Are you performing your day-to-day roles efficiently? If forgetfulness is affecting your work, your role as a parent or grandparent, or any of your other life activities, you may need help.

Above all, says Dr. Berent, know that your memory doesn't have to be perfect to be okay. Some forgetfulness is just part of life.

Think in rhymes. Want to know it? Become a poet. "Make a rhyme for uninteresting things or hard-to-recall facts, or when the information is complicated or highly detailed," says Dr. Herrmann. "Rhymes give us a structure that helps us remember things."

Remember your beta-carotene. Consuming at least one serving daily of foods rich in beta-carotene can improve some aspects of your memory and word fluency or recall, particularly if you're over age 60, according to James G. Penland, Ph.D., research psychologist at the U.S. Department of Agriculture Human Nutrition Research Center in Grand Forks, North Dakota. Dark green vegetables and orange fruits and vegetables are abundant in beta-carotene.

***Observe* rather than *see*.** Seeing something allows for a momentary experience, which may or may not give you the opportunity to soak up details. But observing means paying attention to detail. For instance, you've seen a $20 bill countless times, but can you remember who's pictured on the front of it? Unless you know it's Andrew Jackson, you're not an observer.

"By noticing special properties or features of commonplace items, you will have a better chance to commit them to memory," says psychologist Robin West, Ph.D., of the University of Florida in Gainesville, author of *Memory Fitness over Forty.*

Play mental games. Playing cards or board games like Scrabble is a good way to practice improving your memory, advises Forrest R. Scogin, Ph.D., associate professor of psychology at the University of Alabama in Tuscaloosa. "But choose the games you like, because it can be very frustrating for someone having memory problems to say 'If I just start playing Scrabble, my memory will improve.'" The process is like building up your strength with exercise. Don't expect too much too soon.

To remember names, think of faces. Perhaps the most difficult memory task we're faced with is remembering the names of people we've just met, says Dr. Scogin. The trick is to etch in your mind a permanent association between the name and the face. Better yet, find a prominent feature on the face and focus in on that. If Budd Luzinski, that new guy in the office, happens to have a long nose—visualize a tiny man skiing down that long nose. Imagine that little man losing (Luzinski) those skis.

HANGOVER

Maybe you didn't go so far as to wear the proverbial lamp shade last night. But this morning your head feels as though you wore a streetlight—pole and all. So what do you do now? Here's how to get over that hangover the morning after.

Run for some Gatorade. Even though now is not the time to run a marathon, you can get relief the same way runners do—with Gatorade and other sports drinks that help replace electrolytes (potassium and sodium) and water, says John Brick, Ph.D., biological psychologist and chief of research in the Division of Education and Training at the Center of Alcohol Studies at Rutgers University in New Brunswick, New Jersey. "Part of the problem of being hung over is that you're dehydrated, and beverages like Gatorade replace the essential fluids you lost from drinking." He suggests consuming sports drinks "the morning, afternoon *and* evening after."

Hit the honey. "You can help a hangover by eating a slice of bread or some crackers spread with honey—or any other food that's high in fructose," says Seymour Diamond, M.D., director of the Diamond Headache Clinic in Chicago and executive director of the National Headache Foundation. "That's because fructose [a natural sugar] helps the body burn off alcohol faster, and honey is the sweetener with the highest concentration of fructose." Other good sources of fructose are apples, cherries and grapes.

Have two cups of coffee. "The coffee acts as a vasoconstrictor—something that reduces the swelling of blood vessels that causes headache," adds Dr. Diamond. "A couple of cups can do a great deal to relieve the headaches associated with hangovers." But don't drink too much. You don't need coffee jitters, too.

Get fruit "juiced." A drink may be the last thing you want to reach for now, but relief will come faster if this time you

HOW TO TAKE THE DRUNK OUT OF DRINK

I f you *have* to be a party animal, here are some tips on how to avoid feeling like road kill once the festivities end.

• Nurse your drink. "It sounds obvious, but the slower you drink, the less you drink," says Seymour Diamond, M.D., director of the Diamond Headache Clinic in Chicago and executive director of the National Headache Foundation. "And the less you drink, the less severe your hangover." His advice? Consume no more than one beverage—beer, wine or cocktail—per hour of indulgence.

• Skip the pretzels and nuts. "Salty foods [like those served in most bars] make you thirsty, which makes you drink more," says John Brick, Ph.D., biological psychologist and chief of research in the Division of Education and Training at the Center of Alcohol Studies at Rutgers University in New Brunswick, New Jersey. "The combination of alcohol and salty foods also speeds the dehydrating process, a big factor in hangover."

• Go for protein-rich or high-fat foods. "Cheese and other foods high in protein stay in your digestive system longer, so there's something in your stomach to soak up the alcohol," says Dr. Diamond. The result is a less severe state of intoxication—and thus less of a hangover the next morning.

• Drink "light." Sometimes it's not the alcohol per se that gets you but rather the additives and impurities (called congeners) formed during the making of the beverage. For people sensitive to congeners, a good rule of thumb is the darker the drink, the cloudier your head will feel the next morning, says Dr. Diamond. Vodka doesn't have many congeners, but bourbon, scotch, whisky, red wine and anything aged do.

get juiced on tomato, orange or grapefruit juice. "A large glass of any of these helps in two ways: It's high in fructose, and it's also high in vitamin C, which helps minimize the effects of alcohol," says Dr. Diamond.

Be bullish on bouillon. A bowl or cup of bouillon is the perfect morning-after meal. It's light enough for the way you're feeling, and it can help replenish the salt, potassium and other vitamins and minerals you lose from drinking, says Dr. Diamond.

Have a water nightcap. "The biggest mistake most people make in treating hangovers is not drinking enough water," says Dr. Brick. "Since alcohol is a diuretic that dehydrates the body, I recommend drinking as much as you can before going to bed and then as much as you can the next morning."

Don't take aspirin before you imbibe. Despite popular opinion that taking aspirin *before* you drink will help minimize or avoid a hangover, just the opposite is true. Scientists at the Alcohol Research and Treatment Center at the Veterans Administration Hospital in New York City found that taking aspirin before or during drinking *increases* blood alcohol concentrations to induce a quicker and more severe state of intoxication.

But *do* take it after. If you have a headache or a hangover, you can take aspirin or Alka-Seltzer, but be sure to wait at least four hours after you've finished drinking. "Aspirin is probably still the best way to treat a hangover," says Dr. Brick—but you need to wait a while. Aspirin or similar compounds can be irritating.

Load up on vitamin C. Taking vitamin C before drinking has been shown to counteract some of the effects of alcohol in some people. "In our tests, people who took vitamin C beforehand weren't as severely affected by alcohol as those who didn't take it," says Vincent Zannoni, Ph.D., professor of pharmacology at the University of Michigan in Ann Arbor. "Vitamin C helps by speeding up alcohol clearance from the body."

HEARTBURN

What can you do when that burning sensation right under your rib cage won't go away? You belch. But there's no Ladder Company Number 9 to put out this fire. This is the inferno of that after-dinner bother—heartburn.

The cause of this post-dining fire storm is actually the hard-working sphincter in your lower esophagus. This is a muscle that relaxes to let food pass into your stomach, then quickly closes. But when it doesn't close properly, the contents of your stomach can back up—a condition known as esophageal reflux—creating burning or irritation under your rib cage. Hello, heartburn.

In pregnant women, and in everyone over age 40, the esophageal sphincter is likely to weaken a bit. Not much you can do about that. But the main causes of heartburn are usually obesity, stress and the wrong diet. And those things (unlike age) you *can* do something about.

There's other good news. Your esophagus can heal from the burning caused by stomach acid within seven weeks with proper care, decreasing your chances of recurring episodes. So here's some body-plumbing help that will give your pipes a soothing rest.

Watch out for repeat offenders. Coffee, alcohol, spicy foods and citrus fruits often bring on a five-alarm blaze, according to John Sutherland, M.D., clinical professor of family practice at the University of Iowa College of Medicine in Iowa City and director of the Waterloo Family Practice Residency Program in Waterloo. And watch out for fried and fatty foods as well as tomatoes and chocolate. Any of these can "irritate your esophageal lining or relax your sphincter muscle, triggering reflux," says Ronald L. Hoffman, M.D., director of the Hoffman Center for Holistic Medicine in New York City.

Obliterate that onion. Do you suffer after spicy meals with onions? The onions, not the spices, may be the cause, says Melvin L. Allen, Ph.D., a gastroenterology researcher at the Presbyterian Medical Center of Philadelphia. It also helps to refrigerate raw onions before you slice them. It reduces their potency. Better yet, cook them!

Or opt for a *different* onion. "There are three types of onions that don't cause heartburn," says Stephen Brunton, M.D., director of family medicine at Long Beach Memorial Medical Center in Long Beach, California. "Try the Texas sweet onion, the Maui and the Walla Walla varieties."

Try less on the plate. "Eat small meals to avoid heartburn," advises William J. Ravich, M.D., associate professor of medicine in the Division of Gastroenterology at Johns Hopkins University School of Medicine in Baltimore. It's best to eat more frequent meals of small portions, instead of three "normal" meals a day. And try to have your last meal of the day at least three hours before bedtime, since you're more likely to get heartburn when you're lying down.

Drink water with your meals. Drinking water will wash stomach acids from the surface of the esophagus back into your stomach, says Dr. Hoffman. The saliva you swallow with the water will help neutralize the acid.

Shun the world's worst-for-you dessert. What's the number one food to avoid when you're suffering from heartburn? Chocolate. The sweet confection deals heartburn sufferers a double whammy. It is nearly all fat, *and* it contains caffeine. (For chocolate addicts, however, here's good news: White chocolate, while just as fatty, has little caffeine.)

Four after-dinner no-no's. Your after-dinner habits may be causing your heartburn. For greater comfort, avoid drinking, smoking, napping and strenuous lifting. After-dinner drinks tend to bring on nighttime reflux, Dr. Hoffman says, and "smoking may weaken your lower esophageal sphincter." Avoid lying down after dinner, because gravity helps food stay in your stomach where it belongs. ("Try to resist the after-dinner nap, especially

DON'T FORGET ANTACIDS

Y ou can reach for relief with antacids, but timing is important, says Dennis Decktor, Ph.D., scientific director of the Oklahoma Foundation for Digestive Research in Oklahoma City. "Use antacids after you eat but before heartburn occurs. Food and drink wash them away."

It appears to be the coating action rather than the acid-neutralizing action of antacids that matters, according to Dr. Decktor. For this reason, he advises, "don't drink water with an antacid or you may wash the coating away."

Tablets, pills or liquid? Take a chewable, Dr. Decktor recommends. When you chew, you create saliva, which helps neutralize some of the "burning" acid.

after eating a heavy meal," says Dr. Sutherland.) And as for taking out the garbage after dinner, lifting heavy things after eating can also bring on heartburn, Dr. Ravich says.

Sleep on a slope. "Place the head of your bed on six-inch blocks," advises Dr. Hoffman. "This seems to reduce heartburn by minimizing the flow of reflux from your stomach into your esophagus at night." Also, if you're in the habit of lying on your right side, try sleeping on your left side instead, suggests William B. Ruderman, M.D., chairman of the Department of Gastroenterology at the Cleveland Clinic–Florida in Fort Lauderdale. "The stomach is lower when you're lying on your left side," observes Dr. Ruderman. In that position, stomach acid is less likely to make its way up into your esophagus.

Run not, burn not. Although exercise is a great habit, running can cause "runner's reflux," says Dr. Hoffman. If that's a problem, try other forms of exercise that don't jostle the body as much—such as bicycling or working out with weights. (But avoid any form of exercise except a relaxed stroll right after a meal.)

IT COULD BE AN ULCER

I f you're experiencing heartburn regularly for no apparent reason, it's time to call your doctor, says Samuel Klein, M.D.

How regularly? As a rule of thumb, "two or three times a week for more than four weeks," says Francis S. Kleckner, M.D. Although heartburn is most usually caused by simple acid reflux, he cautions that it can also be a sign of an ulcer.

Heartburn accompanied by any of the following symptoms, says Dr. Klein, should be checked out by a physician *fast.* It could mean you're having a heart attack.

- Difficulty or pain when swallowing.
- Vomiting with blood.
- Bloody or black stool.
- Shortness of breath.
- Dizziness or light-headedness.
- Pain radiating into your neck and shoulder.

In addition, know that heartburn caused by simple acid reflux is normally worse after meals. If your heartburn worsens before meals, it may be a sign of an ulcer.

Review your Rx. Some medications lead to heartburn. For example, "make sure your stomach doctor knows what your heart doctor has prescribed," says John Horn, Pharm.D., associate professor of pharmacy at the University of Washington School of Pharmacy in Seattle. "Certain medications for high blood pressure, particularly calcium channel blockers, can cause reflux."

Try the vomit nut. It's unappealingly named, but the so-called vomit nut, nux vomica, is a homeopathic remedy that relieves heartburn, says Dr. Hoffman. Check your local health food store for availability and follow the directions on the bottle.

HEAT RASH

Sure, the aerobics class was fun, and you worked up a nice sweat. But now it seems you've developed a rash, and your skin feels prickly all the time. Probably both the rash and the pricklies come from sweating—and that means you have heat rash, also known as prickly heat. Heat rash occurs because sweat ducts become plugged and sweat leaks into the skin instead of out of it. But the good news is that it's easy to treat.

How do you know that your rash is prickly heat, as opposed to eczema, an allergic reaction or hives? "If you look at it very closely, you'll see little red dots," says W. Larry Kenney, Ph.D., associate professor of applied physiology at the Laboratory for Human Performance Research at Pennsylvania State University in University Park. "These are sweat glands that have become inflamed at the opening. With further exposure to heat, there will also be a prickly 'pins and needles' sensation on the skin, which is why it is called prickly heat."

Cool off. "Since prickly heat occurs when the sweat ducts are blocked and sweat leaks into the skin, the only way to reverse it is to be in a situation where there is no sweating for a while," says Norman Levine, M.D., chief of dermatology at the University of Arizona College of Medicine Health Sciences Center in Tucson. Cool off, he suggests, by spending as much time as possible in an air-conditioned building for a day or two.

Wear loose clothing. Be selective about the clothing you wear and heat rash may vanish, according to Dr. Kenney. "Anything that will wick moisture away from the body and keep the skin dry will discourage heat rash." Whether you're recovering from heat rash or trying to avoid it, Dr. Kenney suggests that you "choose loose clothing made from cotton or polypropylene and avoid nylon, polyester or any tight-fitting clothes." This is especially important during the summer months.

Wash with mild soaps. To avoid the worst of heat rash, "wash with a mild, antibacterial soap," suggests Rodney Basler, M.D., a dermatologist and assistant professor of internal medicine at the University of Nebraska Medical Center in Omaha. "I would recommend Dial or Lever 2000, followed by a thorough rinsing and drying."

Take a baking soda bath. A baking soda bath can also be beneficial, Dr. Basler says. This will ease the itching and make you feel more comfortable while your heat rash is healing. Just add a few tablespoons of baking soda to your normal bath water and stir it to dissolve completely.

Soothe it with lotion. A number of over-the-counter skin lotions are designed to take the pricklies and itch out of heat rash. Warren Epinette, M.D., a dermatologist at Westwood-Squibb Pharmaceuticals in Buffalo, New York, recommends nonprescription lotions such as Moisturel that contain dimethicone. Calamine, the traditional poison ivy lotion, can also ease the itching and irritation caused by heat rash.

Give it the dust-off. Want to prevent the return of heat rash in hot summer months? Besides wearing loose cotton clothing, you can also dust yourself with absorbent powders. Richard Berger, M.D., clinical professor of dermatology at the University of Medicine and Dentistry of New Jersey Robert Wood Johnson Medical School in New Brunswick, recommends the medicated powder Zeasorb-AF, available in most pharmacies. Cornstarch or talcum powder will also do.

HICCUPS

Hippocrates said that sneezing would bring relief. Plato swore the answer was to hold your breath and gargle. For centuries, the world's greatest minds have pondered long and hard the cures for this most perplexing medical mishap.

Which seems like a real waste of great-mind time. C'mon, we're only talking about *hiccups*, guys.

The *cause* of hiccups is simple: Usually something has triggered involuntary contractions in the diaphragm. You may have swallowed air when you were eating fast or taking a shower or when you suddenly got excited. You can get hiccups from eating an "irritating" food (usually gas inducers such as vegetables or beans) or from eating both hot and cold foods at the same time. Drinking alcohol or carbonated beverages can also set off those involuntary (*hic!*) contractions. In short, just about anything can cause hiccups, says James Lewis, M.D., vice president for medical development at Glaxo Pharmaceuticals in Research Triangle Park, North Carolina, and one of the nation's foremost authorities on hiccup causes and cures.

But whatever the cause, quicker relief is in sight if you:

Hear no evil, have no hiccups. Plugging your ears with your fingers for about 20 seconds can halt hiccups, says Dev Mehta, M.D., a gastroenterologist at Hahnemann University Hospital in Philadelphia. This remedy, reported in the medical journal *Lancet*, operates on the theory that sticking fingers in your ears temporarily short-circuits the vagus nerve, which controls hiccuping. That, in turn, interrupts the hiccup cycle.

Drink pineapple juice . . . or just about anything else. "This is a popular folklore remedy, but we use it in my house when someone gets hiccups, and it works great," says John Renner, M.D., a consumer health expert and clinical professor of family medicine at the University of Missouri at Kansas City. "It's the acidic content of pineapple juice that's said to do the trick, but the truth is, drinking just about any liquid will have the same effect. Drinking requires a lot of swallowing, and doing a lot of swallowing is probably the best way to stop hiccups."

Breathe into a brown paper bag. If swallowing isn't your style, do what the pros do: "The first thing we do when someone comes into the hospital with hiccups is have them breathe into a brown paper bag," says Dr. Mehta. "We're not exactly sure why it works, but we think that breathing more carbon dioxide affects the diaphragm in a way that stops hiccups."

Hold your breath. This age-old remedy really works, says Bahman Jabbari, M.D., chief of neurophysiology in the Department of Neurology at Walter Reed Medical Center in Washington, D.C. "It probably works in the same way breathing into a paper bag does."

Act like a brat. "Sticking your tongue out is another proven remedy," adds Dr. Renner. "It stimulates the glottis, which is the opening of the airway to the lungs"—and a closed glottis causes hiccups.

Rub the roof of your mouth with a cotton swab. It tickles a bit, but Dr. Lewis says it's another way to stimulate the glottis—without looking childish.

INSOMNIA

You think you've got insomnia problems? Pity poor Mrs. Socrates. Seems *Mr.* Socrates, the famed philosopher, had so much trouble getting shut-eye that he would keep his wife up all night—*every* night—expounding his views on the nature of the universe. That is, until one night when she took revenge—by dumping the contents of their chamber pot (the ancient Greeks' version of a toilet) on his head.

That, no doubt, led to further philosophic discussion.

Why are we telling you this? Because if you're cursed with insomnia, you might take some solace in knowing that at least you're in good company. You're sharing this ailment (along with the late, late show) with some 120 million other Americans—among them many hard-driving achievers who can't sleep well because their minds continue to stay active long after their bodies punk out.

If you're among them, don't lose sleep over losing sleep. Here's what you can do to make sure you sleep soundly.

Set a rigid sleep schedule seven days a week. "Sleep is an unavoidable interval in the 24-hour day," says Merrill M. Mitler, Ph.D., director of research for the Division of Chest, Critical Care and Sleep Medicine at the Scripps Clinic and Research Foundation in La Jolla, California. "We insist on people trying to be as regular with their habits as possible."

The key is to get enough sleep so you can make it through your day without drowsiness. To help achieve that goal, try to get to bed at the same time each night so you can set your system's circadian rhythm, the so-called body clock that regulates most internal functions. Just as important is arising at the same time each morning.

Set a sleeping time of, say, 1:00 to 6:00 A.M. If you're sleeping soundly through that 5-hour period, add 15 minutes each week until you get aroused in the middle of the night. Work on getting through that arousal before adding another 15 minutes. You'll know when you reach the point where you've had enough sleep—you'll wake up refreshed, energetic, and ready to take on the day.

If you wake up during the night and can't get back to sleep in

COLOR AWAY INSOMNIA

I f you've tried everything and still have insomnia, maybe you ought to try repainting your bedroom. Why? Because color behaviorists say that color can subconsciously influence our mood, our behavior and even our sleeping patterns.

If that's the case, here are some hues you can use when you decorate for super slumber.

Green evokes peacefulness and serenity and helps lower the heart rate. "Green is comforting to most people and a good color for stress reduction," says color expert Carlton Wagner, director of the Wagner Institute for Color Research in Santa Barbara, California.

Blue is another good choice for the bedroom, since it causes the brain to secrete tranquilizing hormones. "Blue encourages fantasizing and daydreaming," says Wagner.

Violet and other purple shades calm nerves and slow muscular response.

Pink has a calming effect—particularly to the high-strung and easily angered. But different shades appeal to different sexes, says Wagner. "Men prefer yellow-based pinks like apricot and peach, while women go for blue-based pinks like bubble gum."

15 minutes, don't fight it, says Dr. Mitler. Stay in bed and listen to the radio until you're drowsy again.

Again, be sure to wake up at the appointed hour in the morning; don't *sleep in* trying to pick up on "lost" sleep. That goes for the weekends as well. Don't sleep late on Saturday and Sunday mornings. If you do, you may have trouble falling asleep Sunday night, which can leave you feeling washed out on Monday morning.

Take a whiff of lavender. Many people can't fall asleep because they can't relax. But certain smells have been proven to induce a deep sense of relaxation, which can help some people get the shut-eye they need. "A lavender fragrance, for instance, is very effective at inducing a more relaxed state," says Alan R. Hirsch, M.D., a psychiatrist and neurologist who heads the Smell and Taste Treatment and Research Foundation in Chicago. "Other aromas that work very well at lowering stress include spiced apple dishes and other baked desserts as well as the aroma of the salty air of the seashore."

Switch to linen sheets. Researchers at the University of Milan in Italy report that people who sleep on linen sheets fall asleep faster and wake up in a better mood than those using cotton or other fabrics. The researchers believe it may be because linen sheets feel different against the skin and disperse body heat better than other fabrics.

Get a heating blanket (with a timer). "Using a heating blanket will help you get to sleep by relaxing the muscles and increasing brain temperature—two factors that induce sleep," says psychiatrist Henry Lahmeyer, M.D., professor of psychiatry and behavioral sciences at Northwestern University Medical School and co-director of the Sleep Program at Northwestern Memorial Hospital, both in Chicago. "But if you use the blanket all night, you will probably wake up early in the morning. So if you're going to use a heating blanket, use one with a timer, so it will shut off just after you fall asleep."

Try a "white noise" machine. "You can get a white noise machine at Sears or other department stores. The machine emits a sound that helps people get to sleep," adds Dr. Lahmeyer.

Say no to nightcaps. "Alcohol *does* help people get to sleep, but its sleep-inducing effects wear off very quickly. Often people who have taken a nightcap wake up in the middle of the night and then cannot get back to sleep," says Alex Clerk, M.D., director of the Sleep Disorders Clinic at Stanford University in California. "Even when it doesn't cause you to wake up, studies show that alcohol fragments your sleep, so you don't wake up refreshed. A third problem with alcohol as a sleep inducer is that when it's used over time, you develop tolerance, so you need more of it to get to sleep—and that can lead to abuse problems."

Have a midnight snack. If you're having problems hitting the hay, hit the fridge. "A light bedtime snack with protein and sugar increases brain neurotransmitters to induce sleep," says Dr. Lahmeyer. "The classic bedtime snack of a bowl of cereal with milk or a glass of milk with some cookies is perfect." But doctors advise going easy on your noshing, because a heavy meal will disrupt your sleep.

Banish stress. Your bedroom is for sleeping—*period.* (You can make an exception for sex, says psychologist JoyceWalsleben, Ph.D., director of the Sleep Disorders Center at New York University Bellevue Medical Centers.) Too many people turn their bedrooms into offices or rumpus rooms. Instead of sleeping, they're worrying about unpaid bills, disobedient children and tyrannical bosses. No wonder they stay awake! When it's time to pull back the covers, Dr. Walsleben says, you should turn down the day's emotional volume, too.

Table your stress—literally. To get stress makers (kids, bosses, money) off your mind, Dr. Walsleben says, put them on paper. "Write your worries down before you go to bed. That will get them out of your head, and you can tell yourself 'They're on the table, I can worry about them in the morning.'"

JET LAG

Funny thing about air travel: You spend a few hours high in the sky, and you wind up feeling as low as some airline stocks after you land. Blame it on jet lag, that less than uplifting response to time-zone changes that your body doesn't appreciate.

Usually our body clock operates on a 24- to 25-hour cycle that keeps time by stimuli such as eating and sleeping habits, exercise patterns, reactions to light and darkness and other triggers. But when you put yourself in a new time zone—as you do with long-distance travel—you change the normal time of these triggers, which puts your body clock out of sync. The result: headache, earache, fatigue, lethargy, irritability, trouble concentrating and making decisions . . . sometimes even loss of appetite and diarrhea.

And the more time zones you cross, the worse your jet lag. "Basically, the rule of thumb is that after you land, it takes one day to recover for *each* time zone you go through," observes jet lag researcher Charles F. Ehret, Ph.D., senior scientist emeritus at the U.S. Department of Energy Argonne National Laboratory in Argonne, Illinois, and author of *Overcoming Jet Lag.* "So if you're traveling coast-to-coast, that translates to about three days, because you're crossing three time zones," says Dr. Ehret, who is a leading authority on jet lag. "If you cross 15 time zones, as going from New York to Japan may entail, full recovery may take considerably more than a week."

The good news is, you don't *have* to go Greyhound to keep your mood sky-high. Avoiding or remedying jet lag is as easy as making a few minor but significant adjustments in your lifestyle—before leaving, in the air and once you arrive at your destination. Here's how.

Book your flight so that you arrive at night. To help your body adjust to the change in time zones, try to arrange your flights so that you *land* sometime in midevening. That gives you enough time to unwind, eat a good meal and get to bed by 11:00 P.M. *destination time*, says Timothy Monk, Ph.D., associate professor of psychiatry at the University of Pittsburgh School of Medicine and director of the Human Chronobiology Research Program there. Since eastbound travel is most likely to deprive you of adequate shut-eye, researchers at the Royal Air Force Institute of Aviation Medicine in Farnborough, England, suggest this rule: When flying east, fly early; when heading west, fly late.

Avoid in-flight alcohol. Airplane cabins are notoriously dry, and a lengthy trip can dehydrate you faster than a weekend in the Sahara. Dehydration worsens jet lag, and alcohol consumption *worsens* dehydration. "Alcohol is one of the most potent dehydrators there is," says Howie Wenger, Ph.D., an exercise consultant to the globe-trotting Canadian Olympic Team and professional hockey's Los Angeles Kings. Instead of ordering an alcoholic beverage, do what the pros do—load up on fruit juices, water and sports drinks like Gatorade while airborne.

Soak up some sunshine. "One school of thought, and the one I subscribe to, says get out in the sun at your destination as much as possible," says Dr. Monk. The theory, he adds, is that this exposure will help keep your biological clock in the stimulated and awake state during daylight hours at your destination.

"When light strikes the eye, neurotransmitters are released that send an immediate signal to specific regions of the brain," Dr. Ehret explains. "In turn, these brain regions signal the rest of the body that your awake-and-active phase is about to begin."

Make a date with the sun. Some experts feel the time of day you get out in the sunshine is also important. Light earlier in the day appears to shift the body's clock to an earlier hour, while light later in the day seems to shift the body's clock to a later hour, according to Al Lewy, M.D., Ph.D., a psychiatrist at the Oregon Health Sciences University School of Medicine in Portland.

So if you've traveled east, Dr. Lewy suggests getting outside light in the morning. And if you've traveled west, he recommends getting outside light in the afternoon. This only works, however, if you're crossing six or fewer time zones.

Exercise. "It makes sense," Dr. Monk says, "that if you usually go jogging, you should go jogging at your destination. It will get your body pumped up, help alertness and get you out in the sunlight."

A study at the University of Toronto also suggests that exercise will actually reduce the number of days jet lag affects you. Researchers exposed golden hamsters (nocturnal animals with stable activity rhythms) to artificial light and advanced the onset of darkness 8 hours, simulating the conditions of a long flight east.

After darkness, one group of hamsters exercised on a running wheel. The other group mostly slept. While the nonrunning hamsters took 5.4 days to adjust and to resume normal nocturnal activity, the running hamsters adjusted in just 1.6 days.

Do as the Romans do. When you arrive, start adapting to your new environment as quickly as possible. "Get involved—notice the new street names and the language of the people," says Dr. Ehret. "This will help you to adjust."

Socialize. This is especially important if your body is craving sleep, but it's only midafternoon at your destination. "When we're socializing, our bodies assume it's daytime because human beings are, by nature, daytime creatures," says Marijo Readey, Ph.D., a researcher at the Argonne National Laboratory. "That's why many shift workers have symptoms like chronic jet lag."

Don't nap. Or if you do, limit the nap to 1 hour. Napping, Dr. Monk says, will just delay your adjustment to the new time zone.

LACTOSE INTOLERANCE

When you drink a glass of milk, do you bloat up with enough gas to float yourself and Phineas T. Fogg around the world in 80 days? When you eat ice cream, could your subsequent intestinal rumblings substitute for the timpani in the *1812 Overture*? Does a cheese pizza in your belly produce diarrhea in quantities worthy of a laxative study?

If so, you probably have lactose intolerance. That is, your small intestine doesn't produce enough lact*ase*, the enzyme you need to digest lact*ose*, the natural sugar found in dairy products. Never fear, it's not dangerous.

Nor are you alone in your intolerance. The majority of humans get some degree of lactose intolerance by the time they're 20, according to gastroenterologist Seymour Sabesin, M.D., director of the Section of Digestive Diseases at Rush–Presbyterian–St. Luke's Medical Center in Chicago, Illinois. As many as 30 million adult Americans may have some degree of lactose intolerance. But there's good news. You can have your ice cream and eat it, too. Here's how.

Take the tolerance test. Since most everyone's degree of tolerance is different, you'll want to find out how much of a good thing you can have before you stop enjoying it, says Theodore Bayless, M.D., the director of clinical gastroenterology at Johns Hopkins University Hospital in Baltimore.

The obvious thing to do is decrease the amount of milk and dairy products you eat until your symptoms go away.

"Some people are bothered by as little as one-fourth of a glass of milk," he says. "About 30 percent of lactose-intolerant people will get symptoms only after a quart, maybe 30 to 40 percent from a glass."

Put some enzymes in your milk. You don't necessarily have to drink chocolate milk, though. You can simply use enzyme tablets like Lactaid, sold in most drugstores and health food stores. "Even if you're severely lactose-intolerant, you can enjoy milk without any of the symptoms," says Manfred Kroger, Ph.D., professor of food science at Pennsylvania State University in University Park. "Just sprinkle powdered Lactaid into a glass of milk the night before, and the next morning, half the lactose in the milk is gone—and that's enough to prevent any symptoms. Besides, the milk will taste sweeter, because the lactose, which isn't sweet, will break down to glucose, which is."

Eat yogurt. The organisms that make yogurt what it is also produce lactase to digest the lactose contained in yogurt, says Naresh Jain, M.D., a gastroenterologist in private practice in Niagara Falls, New York. "Secondly, the bacteria themselves also probably break down the lactose in the milk. Most people with lactose intolerance don't have it very severely," Dr. Jain says. "Maybe 70 to 80 percent of all otherwise healthy lactose-intolerant people should be able to tolerate yogurt quite well."

Dr. Sabesin notes that "yogurt has only about 75 percent of the lactose content of an equal amount of milk." That difference, Dr. Sabesin says, may be all you need to be able to tolerate lactose. About 4 to 6 ounces a day is about all you need to keep gas away.

LARYNGITIS

You may have lost your voice. But all is not lost. Laryngitis is nature's husky way of saying . . . er, signaling that your vocal cords need a break.

Sometimes extreme hoarseness is the result of a cold or infection, and your voice will return when the cold leaves. Usually, though, laryngitis is more like an injury caused by overusing your vocal cords. Maybe you went for too many high notes in the shower or you rooted for your favorite team a little too enthusiastically. But whether the cause is an infection or a heck-raisin' holler, here's how to rein in the hoarseness and quickly get your voice back to normal.

Don't gargle. A good gargle may seem like an obvious remedy, but it will actually do more harm than good. "Gargling doesn't seem to reach down into the larynx where the irritated or inflamed tissue is," says Robert J. Feder, M.D., a Los Angeles otolaryngologist who teaches singing at the University of Southern California School of Music. "More important, if you make noise as you gargle, the vibration can actually harm inflamed vocal cords."

Stay *completely* quiet. And that means you should avoid whispering, too. It's a given that talking should be avoided: It strains your vocal cords, prolonging or worsening laryngitis. But it's a little-known fact that whispering can be just as bad, or even worse. "Whispering causes you to bang your vocal cords together as strongly as if you were shouting," explains George T. Simpson II, M.D., chairman of the Department of Otolaryngology at the State University of New York at Buffalo School of Medicine and Biomedical Sciences.

Lead your hoarse to water. Downing at least eight glasses of water a day—and preferably ten—ensures that your larynx stays moist, a key step in curing laryngitis. The water should be warm or room temperature—not overly hot or cold. And don't add salt or alcohol. (Forget about hot toddies: They're too drying.) If water isn't your favorite beverage, Dr. Feder says you can also drink juice and warm tea with honey. *Note:* Drink even *more* if you're flying, because the air you breathe in planes is very drying.

Avoid aspirin. If you've lost your voice because you were yelling too loudly, you've probably ruptured a capillary. So stay away from aspirin, advises Laurence Levine, D.D.S., M.D., associate clinical professor of otolaryngology at Washington University School of Medicine in St. Louis. Aspirin increases clotting time, which can impede the healing process.

Choose cough drops wisely. Avoid mint and mentholated products, which are too drying, says Dr. Feder. Stick with honey- or fruit-flavored soft cough drops instead. But keep in mind that cough drops are basically just candy. They don't have any healing effect.

Lubricate with slippery elm. "Slippery elm bark tea is a good lubricant for the back of the throat," says Scott Kessler, M.D., an otolaryngologist in New York City who specializes in performing arts medicine and a physician for many of the performers at the Metropolitan Opera and the City Opera and on Broadway. "Drinking won't lubricate the vocal cords directly. That's because the epiglottis closes over them like a trapdoor. But drinking will provide more water to assist the mucous glands in the larynx to provide a smooth coating on the cords."

Get steamed. Hanging your head over a steaming bowl of water for five minutes two to four times a day can restore lost moisture in your throat and quicken healing time. If you have a cold-air humidifier, that also does the trick, adds Dr. Kessler.

MOTION SICKNESS

T
he sky is blue, the sea is green and you are bright-eyed and rosy-cheeked, out on the deck of a sun-dappled sailboat bobbing along in the waves. Bobbing and dipping. Dipping and lobbing. Lobbing and listing. Listing and rolling. Rolling and rising. Rising and sinking. Sinking and splashing. Splashing and crashing. Crashing and churning. Listing and bobbing and dipping and rippling. Crashing and churning and stomach turning. And before you know it, you're launching your lunch into glistening green waters, quaking and quickening. It's altogether sickening.

The French call it *mal de mer*, and even the most seasoned sailors can suffer from it. In the air, it's airsickness. On land, it's car sickness. And then there's amusement park ride sickness—at least one visitor a day turns green on Disney World's Space Mountain or Big Thunder Mountain roller coaster. But it's all the same thing—that queasy, uneasy feeling collectively known as motion sickness.

"Motion sickness is caused by a conflict between what your eyes tell your brain and what your other senses tell your brain," says Robert M. Stern, Ph.D., professor of psychology at Pennsylvania State University in University Park and a researcher on motion sickness and nausea for the National Aeronautics and Space Administration (NASA). For instance, if you're sitting in the back seat of a car and your eyes are focused on the front seat, your eyes are telling your brain that you're not moving. But there is a part of your inner ear that tells your brain differently. And you feel the bumps on the road; you hear the sounds of passing traffic; you may even smell the fumes. In other words, your senses signal your brain that you *are* moving. It's this mixed message that mixes up your insides. But here's how to remedy the problem.

Don't worry. "Nobody ever died from motion sickness, even though they've felt like they wanted to," says Dr. Stern. "That's important to mention: Anxiety is just going to make you feel worse, because it provokes some of the same undesirable body changes as motion sickness. If you relax and realize this is just a passing thing, you'll fare much better."

Face it on a full stomach. "The biggest mistake people make is not eating, mostly out of fear that if they eat, they will vomit," adds Dr. Stern. "But avoiding food is the worst thing you can do. When you don't eat, the electrical activity of the stomach becomes very unstable, and it's very easy for anything—a bad smell, the sight of another passenger getting sick, whatever—to push you over the boundary and make you vomit. You should eat a small, low-fat meal before traveling, because the stomach is slower to empty fatty foods into the intestines, and you want a meal that will pass through the stomach quickly. And then, while you're traveling, I recommend going no more than two hours without eating something, even if it's just crackers."

Look where you're going. "Being able to look out the window and follow the movement helps a great deal," adds Dr. Stern. "One reason that kids get sick in the back seat of cars so often is that they can't follow the movement of travel. They see only the back of the front seat. Of course, it's easier to watch things go by when you're in a car or boat than in an airplane. But wherever you are, if you're feeling sick, it usually helps just to 'see' where you're going."

Hold your head still. "Minimizing head movements as much as possible can prevent or lessen the effects of motion sickness," says Millard Reschke, Ph.D., senior scientist for sensory function and director of the Neurosensory Lab at NASA in Houston.

Don't read. "Reading is one of the worst things you can do if you suffer from motion sickness—in any mode of transportation, including an airplane," says Dr. Reschke, an expert on motion sickness. (Gee, maybe it's more than coincidence that airlines place those cute little air sickness bags right next to magazines in the seat pocket in front of you.) The reason? Focusing your eyes on the page, rather than the movement, is one way to worsen your condition.

But keep your mind busy. Listening to music, doing problems in your head or other diversionary tactics take the punch out of motion sickness. "That includes doing the driving yourself," says Dr. Stern. "People who usually get motion sickness rarely get it when they drive."

Consider nonprescription medications. Two popular over-the-counter drugs, Dramamine and Bonine, are both effective at preventing motion sickness, but they can cause drowsiness. They're most effective when taken an hour or two before traveling. They can, however, have side effects, so check with your doctor first.

Try ginger for a queasy stomach. For generations, travelers on sailing ships and in bumpy carriages took gingerroot as a cure for nausea. Today, the same motion sickness cure comes in capsules containing the powdered root, and some modern-day travelers find it effective. How much should you take? That depends on how nauseated you are, but "you will know you've had enough when you burp and taste ginger," says Daniel B. Mowrey, Ph.D., a psychologist and psychopharmacologist in Lehi, Utah.

Take the interstate instead. When traveling by car, many people avoid or minimize motion sickness by taking a route *without* a lot of stop-and-go movement.

OILY HAIR

If you've noticed that your hair is oily and you're wondering how it got that way, there are between 90,000 and 140,000 good reasons. That's how many strands of hair are on a reasonably well-covered head, according to Philip Kingsley, a New York City and London hair care specialist. And each strand has its very own oil gland. Strenuous exercise only increases oil production, as do heat and humidity. Plus there's pollution. And hormones. And sweat. And residue from all those hair products you may have used to control the oiliness.

It goes for anyone: If you've got a full head of hair and live a relatively active life, then some extra oil is almost inevitable. But hair color does make some kind of difference, adds Kingsley. Redheads with thick, coarse hair, for example, rarely have problems with oily hair, while blondes with silky, baby-fine hair have the worst problem. (So much for having more fun!)

But whatever your hair color or the problems with your hair, here's how to ease the oiliness.

Choose the right shampoo. The obvious answer to oily hair is to shampoo often—daily is recommended by most of our experts. But if you're using the wrong shampoo, you could be disappointed with the results. "Look for a shampoo that's designated as 'deep cleaning' and for other descriptions on the packaging that indicate the shampoo cleanses well," suggests John Corbett, Ph.D., vice president of technology for Clairol, based in Stamford, Connecticut.

"Clear, see-through shampoos tend to have less goo in them," adds Thomas Goodman, Jr., M.D., assistant professor of dermatology at the University of Tennessee Center for Health Sciences in Memphis. "They clean away oil more effectively and don't leave a residue."

And use it the right way. Most often recommended is a double shampoo, leaving the suds on your head for *at least* five minutes each time, says Lowell Goldsmith, M.D., professor and chairman of the Department of Dermatology at the University of Rochester School of Medicine and Dentistry in Rochester, New York. (If your head isn't especially oily, a single shampoo is enough, as long as you leave the shampoo on for the full five minutes.)

Take a powder. "If your hair is oily after a difficult, tense day, I suggest you do a temporary 'dry' shampoo by sprinkling a tiny amount of talcum powder onto your hair one section at a time. Rub the powder first onto the scalp, then through the hair with your fingers," says Karen E. Burke, M.D., Ph.D., a dermatologist and dermatologic surgeon in New York City. "The powder very effectively absorbs some of the oil." But be careful not to use too much powder or your hair will look white and dull, and you may even have difficulty with static electricity, making your hair difficult to style.

Rinse your hair with vinegar. One teaspoon of apple cider kitchen vinegar added to a pint of water makes an excellent finishing rinse that adds shine and luster to your hair while removing soap residue that can weigh down oily hair. A thorough rinsing with plain water will remove the smell.

Or freshen it with lemon. Squeezing the juice of two lemons into a pint of distilled water makes another excellent rinse that helps cut oiliness, adds David Daines, owner of David Daines Salon in New York City.

OILY SKIN

Maybe your forehead shines a little. Okay, so maybe it shines *a lot.* There are many reasons for a facial gloss that resembles 10W-40 motor oil: hormones (particularly when you're pregnant), stress, the cosmetics you use and *especially* heredity.

But before you start chopping down your family tree, know there's some good news. Just as it protected your ancestors against the harsh weather, that excess oil can protect your skin from Father Time, helping you age more gracefully and wrinkle less than those with dry or normal skin.

Still, promises of future youth may not convince you to accept the oil of today. So if you want to change things a bit oil-wise, here's how.

Give your face a "tea" steam bath. "A good treatment for oily skin is to steam the face using some Swiss Kriss herbal laxative. Make a 'tea' by boiling about two tablespoons of Swiss Kriss in a big spaghetti pot filled with about two to three quarts of water," says Karen E. Burke, M.D., Ph.D., a dermatologist and dermatologic surgeon in New York City. "After you take the pot off the stove, place your head over the steam for about one to three minutes, then rinse your face with cold water." Doing this about once or twice each week opens pores and removes excess oils, says Dr. Burke. Swiss Kriss is sold in many health food stores.

Go synthetic. Oily skin should be cleansed at least twice daily, but use your fingertips, not stiff washcloths or polyester scrubs, advises Nelson Lee Novick, M.D., associate clinical professor of dermatology at Mount Sinai School of Medicine in New York City. Use sensitive-skin cleansers labeled "synthetic," he suggests. The synthetic cleansers won't leave scummy deposits on your skin, as regular soap can. (The deposits can further clog your pores and contribute to oiliness.)

Follow with astringents. Astringents with acetone are your best bet, according to Kenneth Neldner, M.D., a professor and chairman of the Department of Dermatology at the Texas Tech University Health Sciences Center School of Medicine in Lubbock. "Acetone is a great fat and grease solvent, and most astringents have a bit of acetone in them. If you use it regularly, you can surely remove oil from the skin."

Although most astringents contain alcohol, look for a brand that also contains acetones, such as Seba-Nil, says Dr. Neldner. Ordinary rubbing alcohol, however, can be used as an effective, inexpensive astringent. Those looking for something milder can try witch hazel, which contains some alcohol and also works well.

Nonalcohol astringents contain mostly water and are not as effective as those with alcohol and acetone, but they may be of help for those with sensitive skin. Worth noting: Dermatologists say that rather than washing the face several times a day, which can leave it too dry and irritated, you're better off to carry astringent pads with you and use them to cleanse the face.

Mask yourself in mud. Clay or mud masks—available at most stores where beauty products are sold—offer temporary relief, adds Howard Donsky, M.D., associate professor of medicine at the University of Toronto, and author of *Beauty Is Skin Deep.* Generally, the darker the color of the mud, the more oil it will absorb. White or rose-colored clays are best suited for sensitive skin.

Wipe yourself clean. If you have exceptionally oily skin, you can remove oil from your skin by gently blotting your face with soft tissues, advises dermatologist Michael Ramsey, M.D., clinical instructor of dermatology at Baylor College of Medicine in Houston.

Cast the witch hazel spell. For extra punch, dab a little witch hazel on the tissues—it's one of the most effective oil absorbers for the money, according to Dr. Burke.

Wash with hot water. Using hot water when you wash your face dissolves skin oil more effectively than using cool or tepid water, says Hillard H. Pearlstein, M.D., assistant clinical professor of dermatology at Mount Sinai School of Medicine in New York City.

Take a lesson from your child. The same products that teenagers use to clean their faces during those traumatic "acne years" are effective on your oily skin. (After all, acne is caused by clogged oil glands, among other factors.) When shopping, look for benzoyl peroxide gel, preferably in a low-strength (2.5 percent) formulation, to minimize potential irritation.

Select cosmetics with care. "Cosmetics come in two major categories," says Dr. Neldner, "oil-based and water-based. If you've got oily skin, use only water-based products."

There are many cosmetics formulated for oily skin. They are made to soak up and cover oiliness so the skin doesn't look as greasy. But no cosmetic has any magical ingredient that will slow down or stop oil production, so don't be lured into buying products that make such claims.

PAPER CUTS

The pen is mightier than the sword"—at least according to playwright Baron Edward Bulwer-Lytton. But slice your finger on the edge of an innocent-looking piece of paper and . . . *yowwwwwww*! You'll learn firsthand of the awesome power of office supplies.

But here's what you can do about this skin-deep slice of life.

Use glue to renew. It's not exactly the kind of stuff they teach in medical school, but Krazy Glue, Super Glue or any other clear, super-strength bonder offers the fastest relief known to modern medicine. "It's really the best thing there is," says Rodney Basler, M.D., a dermatologist and assistant professor of internal medicine at the University of Nebraska Medical Center in Omaha. "It eliminates pain in about three seconds, because it immediately stops the air from hitting nerve endings—and air touching the nerves is what causes the pain. Just place a drop on the cut and repeat it the following day."

Although it "seals" instantly, a drop of this glue wears off in a day or so. Just be sure you don't touch something in the instant or so before it dries, because it does bond very quickly to whatever you touch.

Adds Nelson Lee Novick, M.D., associate clinical professor of dermatology at Mount Sinai School of Medicine in New York City: "These glues plasticize so quickly that they act as a sealant, so healing can take place while the finger is protected from air and germs. And they're completely safe, because a paper cut is so minor that they never enter the bloodstream." However, Elmer's and other white and yellow glues don't work this way.

Apply New-Skin. "A product called New-Skin, available at your drugstore, stings a little but acts as a liquid dressing and is excellent for paper cuts," says Dr. Novick.

Feel serene with Vaseline. If you have no super-strength bonder or antibiotic ointment, apply some petroleum jelly (Vaseline) to the cut. "It acts as a coating that prevents air from getting to sensitive, exposed tissue," says Dr. Basler. "It also provides a moist base, so new skin tissues can grow more easily than if you apply nothing."

Nail that pain with nail polish. In a pinch, dabbing some clear nail polish *after* cleaning the wound will also seal it against air and germs, adds Dr. Novick. However, it doesn't promote faster healing.

Take the boo-hoo out of boo-boos. For deep cuts, the problem isn't putting on an adhesive strip, it's taking it off. To remove adhesive strips without stripping your skin, use nail scissors to separate the gauze part in the center from the adhesive, says Dr. Novick. Lift off the gauze center, then gently pull the adhesive strips from your skin on either side.

POISON PLANTS

Who else but prolific Mother Nature could provide us with itches in triplet form—poison ivy, oak and sumac? These three plants are annoying as all outdoors to an estimated 50 million people each year. At least half the U.S. population has some allergic reaction to this trio. In fact, this is the most common allergy known to humans.

The wicked itch and bothersome rash of these "poisons" are caused by urushiol oil, a light, colorless or slightly yellow oil, one of the world's most potent toxins. A mere one-billionth of a gram is enough to cause sensitive folks to scratch themselves silly. And far more than one-billionth is released whenever the plant is "bruised," which happens *any* time there is direct contact with the leaves, stems or roots.

The potency of urushiol oil lasts about five years, so you can get a reaction from handling unwashed garden tools that were used to dig up poison ivy years earlier. But the oil does wash away. So if you wash yourself and your garden tools with soap and water within 15 minutes after contact, you can help avoid a later rash. Applying calamine lotion and taking oatmeal baths are probably the best-known cures once you've been exposed, but here are some other ways to rush the rash and nix Mother Nature's mother of all itches.

Have a milk soak. "A compress with ice-cold milk helps dry the rash and soothe the itch," says John F. Romano, M.D., a dermatologist and clinical assistant professor of medicine at The New York Hospital–Cornell Medical Center in New York City. "Just soak milk in gauze and apply it to your skin." *Note:* Whole milk seems to work; skim milk doesn't have the same effect, though doctors aren't sure why. Also, since milk can leave skin smelling "sour," be sure to rinse yourself off with cool water after each application.

Rub on baking soda. "If your rash is blistering or weeping, make a paste of water and baking soda and apply it to the skin," advises dermatologist Rodney Basler, M.D., assistant professor of internal medicine at the University of Nebraska Medical Center in Omaha. "This helps dry up the oozing blisters." If the area itches without blistering, however, the baking soda paste won't have much effect.

Enlist help from M.O.M. "Although it's not made for this purpose, milk of magnesia can relieve poison ivy itch as well as calamine lotion," says Dr. Romano. That's because anything alkaline usually helps relieve itch, and milk of magnesia is alkaline. And since it's a thinner solution than calamine, it's easier to apply, Dr. Romano points out.

Try a dose of deodorant. The U.S. Forestry Service asked William Epstein, M.D., professor of dermatology at the University of California, San Francisco, School of Medicine, to come up with an inexpensive way to protect forest rangers from poison ivy. He found an unusual answer: spray deodorant. Aluminum chlorohydrate and other agents in spray deodorants prevent oils in poison ivy from irritating the skin. So in a pinch, spraying arms and legs with a deodorant can help protect you. But Dr. Epstein notes that there are commercial products that work better.

Stop the itch with ice. "By far the cheapest effective remedy once you have contracted poison ivy is to apply an ice cube to the affected area for about one minute," says Dr. Romano. "The ice cools the itch." If you don't have any ice cubes, it helps to run cold water over the areas.

Zap it with zinc. Although it's not the most effective choice, zinc oxide, according to some experts, helps soothe itching and may help dry the rash. An inexpensive, over-the-counter skin ointment best known as the stuff lifeguards wear on their noses, zinc oxide is one of the active ingredients in calamine lotion.

Learn not to burn. Don't try to rid your backyard of poison ivy by burning it. That releases droplets of urushiol oil,

A RASH OF RUMORS

Misconceptions about poison ivy, oak and sumac are almost as widespread as the plants. Let's set the record straight.

- Myth: Poison ivy is contagious. Fact: Rubbing the rashes won't spread poison ivy to other parts of your body (or to another person). You spread the rash only if urushiol oil—the sticky, resinlike substance that causes the rash—has been left on your hands.
- Myth: You can get poison ivy simply by being near the plants. Fact: Direct contact is needed to release urushiol oil.
- Myth: Leaves of three, let them be. Fact: Poison sumac has 7 to 13 leaves on a branch, although poison ivy and oak have 3 leaves per cluster.
- Myth: Don't worry about dead plants. Fact: Urushiol oil stays active on any surface, including dead plants, for up to five years.

which can be inhaled and cause serious damage to your lungs. Instead, dig it up—roots and all—and dispose of it in a sealed container. Then wash yourself, your clothes and your tools thoroughly.

Go commercial. To help prevent another attack, there are several over-the-counter poison ivy repellents such as Ivy Shield, which is sold in most drugstores.

POSTNASAL DRIP

Some mucus is always gliding effortlessly down the back of your throat, but what happens when that normal trickle turns into Chinese mucus torture—the steady drip you know (and dread) as *postnasal*?

You hack. You ahem. You swallow. You snort.

In short, you suffer.

Some causes of postnasal drip are well known, such as colds and allergies. A less recognized cause is aging, when mucus turns a bit thicker and more obtrusive. So much for the causes. How about the cures?

Squirt in some salt and soda. Saline sprays or drops will help flush away excess nasal secretions, says Gailen D. Marshall, Jr., M.D., Ph.D., assistant professor and director of the Allergy and Clinical Immunology Division at the University of Texas Medical School in Houston. In eight ounces of water, dissolve ¼ teaspoon of table salt and ¼ teaspoon of baking soda. Use a nosedropper to squirt about half of the solution up your nose, he advises.

Give your throat a saline swish. Once you've rinsed out your nostrils, gargle with the remainder of the saline solution. "That will soothe a scratchy throat and help eliminate the drainage sensation," Dr. Marshall says.

Water down your woes. "You want to keep that mucus as thin as possible," says Alexander C. Chester, M.D., clinical professor of medicine at Georgetown University Medical Center in Washington, D.C. Steaming your nose in a hot shower or sauna, drinking a lot of water and humidifying the air will lighten the load on your nose and throat, he says.

Blow your nose regularly. This may be so obvious that you overlook it, says Jerald Principato, M.D., an otolaryngologist in private practice in Bethesda, Maryland, and associate clinical professor of otolaryngology at George Washington University

School of Medicine. The simple act of blowing eliminates some excessive postnasal drainage from the front of the nose.

Get a rise out of lying down. If you notice the sensation of secretions in your throat at night, try raising the head of the bed by putting a few books under the legs of the headboard. (Be sure the bed will remain steady.) The drip won't pool in the back of your throat, and any stomach contents that might be creeping up your throat will drain back to where they belong, says Mark Loury, M.D., assistant professor in the Department of Otolaryngology and Head and Neck Surgery at Johns Hopkins University Hospital in Baltimore.

Don't scoff at a cough cure. Over-the-counter anticough preparations such as Robitussin and Vicks Formula 44 also thin the mucus, says Horst R. Konrad, M.D., chairman of the Division of Otolaryngology and Head and Neck Surgery at Southern Illinois University School of Medicine in Springfield. These preparations will at least allow your mucus to take a smoother ride down your throat.

Turn on the humidifier. A good humidifier, one that takes several gallons of water to fill, can help keep your nasal passages moist during the dry winter months. And this can help keep mucus from drying out and getting so thick you notice it.

RESTLESS LEGS SYNDROME

Scientists call this condition Ekbom syndrome, RLS or nocturnal jerking movements—and if you're a sufferer, the poor schmoe you sleep with probably has a few choice monikers for it, too. That's because when your restless legs start running at night, you're likely to give your bedmate a swift kick or two as your legs thrash about seeking nightly relief.

But what makes them restless? Maybe your legs seek relief from a cramplike feeling. Or perhaps your thighs feel as though bugs were crawling inside them. Sometimes the pain is deep and throbbing. Other times it feels like pins and needles. The feelings vary but not the scenario: During periods of rest—especially as you're going to sleep—your legs get antsy, and moving them is the action that brings relief. And it's not just legs and feet, either—your hands may go through those nightly motions as well.

One in 20 Americans has restless legs syndrome, which may be inherited. Doctors believe it may be triggered by stress, a nutritional deficiency or some sort of imbalance in brain chemistry. It is not dangerous and doesn't lead to serious neurological disorders. In fact, many doctors think restless legs syndrome is an annoyance rather than a bona fide disease. But here's how to get a leg up on restless legs.

Exercise before bedtime. "People report that if they exercise sometime during the day, they are less likely to be bothered by restless legs at night. For best results, I recommend that you do deep knee bends or other leg exercises as close to bedtime as possible," suggests Arthur S. Walters, M.D., associate professor of neurology at the University of Medicine and Dentistry of New Jersey Robert Wood Johnson Medical School in New Brunswick and a researcher into the causes and cures of restless legs syndrome.

Since leg exercises or taking a walk brings only short-term relief, Dr. Walters stresses that you need to exercise close to the time when you're going to bed. Exercise helps by releasing endorphins, the body's natural painkilling substances that may ease restless legs symptoms.

Take your vitamins. Several studies have shown that iron deficiency can trigger symptoms of restless legs syndrome. Others blame a folate deficiency. To cover all the bases, take a multivitamin/mineral supplement every day to protect yourself against both deficiencies and possibly against restless legs, advises Lawrence Z. Stern, M.D., professor of neurology and director of the Mucio F. Delgado Clinic for Neuromuscular Disorders at the University of Arizona College of Medicine Health Sciences Center in Tucson.

Stop smoking. "It's certainly worth trying," says Janet A. Mountifield, M.D., a general practitioner in Toronto, who noticed that one of her patients was cured of restless legs syndrome after quitting a longtime smoking habit. One possible theory: Smoking impairs blood flow to leg muscles. "I don't know if it was a fluke, but my patient tried everything. Nothing worked for her restless legs—until she quit smoking."

Sip the grape. Douglas K. Ousterhout, M.D., D.D.S., clinical professor of surgery (plastic) at the University of California, San Francisco, and a former restless legs sufferer, says he relieved his symptoms (as well as his mother's) simply by drinking wine. "Ever since I started to drink a glass of wine each night, I've never had a problem," he says. His mother also got over restless legs syndrome by having a glass or two a week. Although Dr. Ousterhout initially thought that red wine did the trick, "I've since learned that white wine works just as well—although I can't think of any scientific explanation and have no idea why it works."

Soak your feet. A cool-water soak just before bedtime is a good way to chill restless leg pain. "Many people soak their feet in cool water, and it seems to help somewhat, so I think it's worth trying," says Ronald F. Pfeiffer, M.D., associate professor of neurology and pharmacology at the University of Nebraska Medical Center in Omaha. Just don't overdo it. Immersing feet in ice or extremely cold water can cause nerve damage, so keep the water at least 50°F.

Or massage your legs. "Rubbing your legs briskly, or running a vibrator over them, also brings relief for many people," says Dr. Pfeiffer. Many experts believe it's because massaging can "shut off" the pain impulses caused by restless legs.

Don't eat a big meal late. "It may be the activity of the nervous system involved in digesting a big meal that triggers symptoms," offers Dr. Stern.

And don't drink coffee at all. Some studies show that eliminating caffeine from your diet can bring relief. "In general, stimulants can aggravate restless legs syndrome in some people, and getting rid of stimulants such as coffee can relieve symptoms," adds Dr. Pfeiffer.

Take a jolt. Don't be alarmed if your doctor sends you home with a rented black box and instructions to plug yourself in. Some researchers believe that TENS treatments—*TENS* stands for transcutaneous electrical nerve stimulation—can significantly relieve the symptoms of restless legs. With TENS, electrodes are placed on the skin over the affected parts of your legs. Small amounts of electricity then are directed into the underlying muscles and nerves. Essentially, your legs become too distracted by the electricity to continue being restless.

SNORING

There are different levels of snoring. "If your wife moves out of the bedroom, then you snore at a moderate level," says Philip Westbrook, M.D., director of the Mayo Clinic Sleep Disorders Center in Rochester, Minnesota. "But if your neighbors move, then you're a heavy snorer."

Snoring is often caused by gravity acting on loose tissue in the upper airway, says Peter Hauri, Ph.D., co-director of the Mayo Clinic Sleep Disorders Center in Rochester, Minnesota. When you're lying on your back, either the tissue or your tongue "falls" into your throat and obstructs your airway.

Go on a diet. Most snorers tend to be middle-aged, overweight men. Most women snorers are past menopause. Slimming stops snoring. "Snoring is frequently related to being overweight," says Earl V. Dunn, M.D., a professor of family medicine and a researcher at the University of Toronto Sunnybrook Medical Centre Sleep Laboratory. "We've found that if a moderate snorer loses weight, the snoring becomes less loud, and in some people it actually disappears."

"You don't have to be a 2-ton Tony to develop snoring. Just being a little overweight can bring on a problem," says Philip Smith, M.D., director of the Johns Hopkins University Sleep Disorders Center in Baltimore. "Men about 20 percent over ideal body weight can develop snoring. Women have to be much heavier, usually 30 to 40 percent over ideal body weight. But the more overweight you are, the more likely it is that your airway will collapse."

Ignore the midnight spirits. "Alcohol before bed makes snoring worse," says Dr. Dunn. Don't drink and sleep.

Stay away from sedatives. Sleeping pills may make you sleep, but they will keep your partner awake. "Anything that relaxes the tissues around the head and neck will tend to make snoring worse. Even antihistamines will do it," says Dr. Dunn.

Snooze on your side or stomach. It's no coincidence that most problem snorers sleep on their backs. "Basically, when you're on your back, your tongue falls back like a wet rag into your throat," says Bernard DeBerry, M.D., a Laguna Hills, California, surgeon who specializes in procedures related to snoring and sleep apnea and who is clinical associate professor of surgery in the Head and Neck Division at the University of California, Irvine, College of Medicine. "That's not exactly helpful in maintaining a clear airway." That's why *all* experts say sleeping in another position—preferably on your stomach—usually helps decrease both the volume and incidence of snoring.

Get more sleep. "It's not a well-known fact, but sleep loss causes snoring," says Thomas Roth, Ph.D., president of the National Sleep Foundation and director of the Henry Ford Hospital Sleep Disorders and Research Center in Detroit. "If you're snoring and not sleeping enough, you may be able to fix the problem by going to bed an hour or so earlier or sleeping later."

Sleep on a firm mattress. If your mattress is soft or saggy, get a new firm one. A flat, firm mattress helps keep your neck straight and reduces obstructions in your airway, according to Portland, Oregon, otolaryngologist Derek S. Lipman, M.D., author of *Stop Your Husband from Snoring*.

Exercise regularly. "People who exercise regularly are much less likely to form congestion in the upper respiratory tract," says Dr. DeBerry. Besides, regular aerobic exercise improves cardiovascular health and strengthens overall breathing and lung capacity, which may offset problems that lead to snoring. But exercise should be avoided just before bedtime, since it can "leave your body too charged up to sleep," he adds.

STRESS

I f you've been sick lately, suspect stress. Some doctors say that as many as *nine of ten* visits to the doctor may be related to stress. That includes everything from allergies and asthma to herpes and heart disease.

Now if that little bit of news isn't stressing enough, there's also those angst-inducing traffic jams, long lines and inept workers. And let's not forget unemployment, pollution, crime and your home's lousy plumbing.

If all these small annoyances and big frustrations push your stress button, it's worth doing something about, because uncontrolled stress can lead to burnout—that dragged-out, done-in feeling that you just can't move ahead or get anything done. Although "job burnout" is the common phrase, when stress goes wild, your health and home life as well as your work are affected.

But instead of staying burned up and burned out, why not try some of the tactics experts recommend for staying cool?

"Audit" your stress. To control stress, you have to first determine what *is* the stress in your life, says Paul J. Rosch, M.D., clinical professor of medicine and psychiatry at New York Medical College in Valhalla and president of the American Institute of Stress in Yonkers. "To do that, sit down and list *all* the things in your life you find especially stressful. Then separate them into two categories: things you can do something about, and those you cannot control and must learn to accept." This process will enable you to allocate your time where it'll do the most good—and to stop worrying about things you can't do anything about.

Look for the silver lining. "The key to controlling stress is to monitor and challenge your negative thinking," says psychologist Richard Blue, Ph.D., a stress management specialist with the Behavioral Institute of Atlanta. "When you look for the positive side of what's causing you stress—and usually you *can* find some positive things about it—you'll see that it's probably not as stressful as you're making it out to be."

To train yourself to think more positively, begin each sentence with "at least" whenever you're stressed out, advises Dr. Blue. *Examples*: If you work for a jerky boss, remind yourself "At least I have a job." When you're stressed out because of a leaky kitchen faucet, tell yourself "At least I own a house."

Reevaluate your role in life. "In most cases, stress burn-out is the result of a mismatch between your personality or goals and the realities of a situation," says Dr. Rosch. That means asking yourself some hard questions and giving yourself honest answers—about your work ethic, talents and true desires. "Find the right match between your job and your personality and the odds are you'll never suffer job burnout," says Dr. Rosch.

Rate your responses. "Most of our stress is the result of 'catastrophizing,'" says Allen Elkin, Ph.D., a practicing psychologist and program director at the Stress Management and Counseling Center in New York City. One way to stop catastrophizing is to rate the importance of your stressor on a simple 1 to 10 scale. If you miss the subway, you may give yourself a 4; if you lose your wallet, an 8. Then think of some *real* stressors—a heart attack, losing a job, a death in the family—and go back and rerate the missed subway and lost wallet. "Over time, you'll recognize when you're catastrophizing situations and get some more balance," says Dr. Elkin.

Take a Zen-second relaxation break. "One thing that's very effective at helping with stress is a method I call rapid relaxation, which takes about 10 or 20 seconds," says Dr. Elkin. "You take a deep breath, deeper than normal, and hold it in until you notice a little discomfort. At the same time, squeeze your thumb and first finger together, as if you were making the okay sign, for six or seven seconds. Then exhale slowly through your mouth, release the pressure in your fingers, and allow all your tension to drain out.

"Repeat these deep breaths three times to extend the relaxation. With each breath, allow your shoulders to droop, your jaw to drop and your body to relax. I recommend doing this several times throughout the day, particularly when you begin to feel stress building."

Soak yourself. A warm—*not* hot—bath helps reduce stress by increasing peripheral circulation and relaxing muscles, which causes a calming effect. Soak for no more than 15 minutes in water 100° to 102°F. This is an effective time and temperature for stress relief.

Get a pet. Research by Alan Beck, Sc.D., professor of ecology at Purdue University School of Veterinary Medicine in West Lafayette, Indiana, and author of *Between Pets and People*, shows that when people pet an animal, their blood pressure, heart rate and *stress* drop almost immediately. "I think one reason is because touching an animal is one of the few socially acceptable opportunities for many people to show outward affection—and people *do* have a need for touch.

"Even looking at fish in an aquarium has similar effects. The eyebrows become less furrowed, there's a more relaxed smile and sometimes even a slight drooping of the eyes—all facial expressions that indicate being at ease and less stressed," he says.

Stretch your body. "Stretching can help you feel more peaceful and relaxed," says Dean Ornish, M.D., director of the Preventive Medicine Research Institute in Sausalito, California, and author of *Dr. Dean Ornish's Program for Reversing Heart Disease.* Whenever you get a break during the day, do some easy stretches. "Just as your mind affects your body, your body can affect your mind," says Dr. Ornish. He suggests that you practice your stretches with slow, fluid movements. (And wear loose, comfortable clothing that *allows* you to stretch easily.)

Press your head. Applying light pressure on your temples with a circular motion helps massage nerves, which in turn relaxes muscles throughout your body, says Emmett Miller, M.D., medical director of the Cancer Support and Education Center in Menlo Park, California.

POSITIVE THOUGHTS, POSITIVE FEELINGS

Thoughts cause feelings, and the wrong kinds of thoughts can cause stressful feelings. "We cause ourselves a lot of unnecessary anxiety by seeing the glass as half empty rather than as half full," says Fran Gaal, a psychotherapist in Bethlehem, Pennsylvania.

Do you automatically interpret silence on the part of your spouse to mean anger when it could just as easily mean fatigue? Do you blame yourself when a sudden downpour drenches your wash on the line? Do you dwell on the few times your boss criticized your performance and ignore the innumerable times she's praised you?

We all fall into the negative thinking rut from time to time. We badger ourselves with "should haves" and lose sight of the fact that "good" and "bad" in life is rarely black and white.

"Think in shades of gray," recommends psychiatrist and cognitive therapist David Burns, M.D., "not black or white only." All-or-nothing thinking can lead to anxiety, depression, feelings of inferiority, perfectionism and anger. Allow yourself to fail now and then. It's all part of being human.

Have a good cry. It's one of the oldest and most effective responses to stress—and it still works as well now as when Adam and Eve shed a tear over the stress of buying a new home. Not only crying but yelling and other emotional outbursts may help release pent-up frustration and stress, says Dr. Miller. But choose wisely where to yell—in an auto works well.

Sunburn

Even before there was a hole in the ozone layer, going to the seashore could leave you sea-sore. But now, with more harmful ultraviolet rays peeking through, limiting your sun exposure is essential, particularly between the sizzling summer hours of 10:00 A.M. and 3:00 P.M. The best prevention is also a wise precaution: Wear sunscreen with an SPF (sun protection factor) of 15 *all* the time.

Okay, but maybe you forgot. And now you're in pain. Well, you can try those old standbys aloe and over-the-counter hydrocortisone cream. Even an extra moisturizer can help a lot. But when you have too much fun in the sun, here are some *other* ways to take the fire out of sunburn pain.

Just add milk. "Dip some gauze into milk and apply it to your sunburned skin," says dermatologist John F. Romano, M.D., clinical assistant professor of medicine at The New York Hospital–Cornell Medical Center in New York City. The milk should be about room temperature or slightly cooler but not refrigerator-cold. "Milk is an excellent remedy for any kind of burn," notes Dr. Romano.

Keep this milk compress on the burn for 20 minutes or so, and repeat every two to four hours. Since milk can leave skin smelling "sour," be sure to rinse yourself off with cool water afterward.

Be soothed by vegetables. Boil some lettuce in water, then strain it and let the liquid cool for a few hours in the refrigerator before applying it to your skin with cotton balls, recommends Lia Schorr, a New York City skin care specialist and author of *Lia Schorr's Seasonal Skin Care.* Other vegetables that produce results? Thinly sliced pieces of raw cucumber, potato or apple can be placed on sunburned areas such as the forearm. The coolness from the vegetables is soothing and might help reduce inflammation.

Get Jolly Green skin care. Wrapping a bag of frozen corn or peas in a towel and applying it to the burned area also helps cool the pain, says dermatologist Frederic Haberman, M.D., a clinical instructor of medicine at Albert Einstein College of Medicine of Yeshiva University in the Bronx. But be sure to wrap it first, so you don't place the icy package directly on your skin.

Double your dosage of pain reliever. "Probably the best thing you can do is to take *two times* the recommended amount of ibuprofen or another pain reliever for the first two doses and then go to the recommended dose," advises Dr. Romano. Doubling the usual dosage of ibuprofen or aspirin helps block a chemical in your body that causes pain. But check with your doctor, since some people have a reaction to aspirin.

Eat for vitamin E. A regular dose of vitamin E is thought to do a host of good, providing protection from a variety of things from heart attack in men to fibroid tumors in women. "It also decreases the inflammation you can get from sunburn," says Karen E. Burke, M.D., Ph.D., a dermatologist and dermatologic surgeon in New York City who has studied the effects of vitamin E. Good food sources of vitamin E include whole grains such as wheat germ, vegetable oils—especially sunflower and soybean oil—and nuts.

If you choose to purchase vitamin E supplements, be sure to read the small print: You should get only the natural form. But check with your doctor before taking vitamin E or other vitamin supplements.

What about rubbing vitamin E on your skin? Although you can also treat sunburn with a direct application of vitamin E by opening a vitamin E acetate capsule and rubbing the liquid directly on your skin, it's more effective to take it internally to decrease sunburn pain, suggests Dr. Burke.

Soak yourself in diluted vinegar. "Pour one cup of white kitchen vinegar into a tub of tepid water and soak yourself in it," advises Harry Roth, M.D., clinical professor of dermatology at the University of California, San Francisco. "It's very soothing to your skin and helps relieve the pain of sunburn."

Or try baking soda and cornstarch. Another recipe for relief, also from the kitchen cabinet: Mix ¼ cup of baking soda and ¼ cup of cornstarch into a tub of tepid water and soak yourself, adds Dr. Roth.

Heal with oatmeal. If you find the smell of vinegar or milk too intense, you can wrap dry oatmeal in some gauze or cheesecloth and run cool water through it, suggests Dr. Haberman. Wring out the excess water and apply the cloth for 20 minutes every two to four hours.

Don't be *too* clean. While you have sunburn, stay away from highly fragrant bubble baths, soaps, colognes and perfumes, says Thomas Gossel, Ph.D., R.Ph., professor of pharmacology and toxicology at Ohio Northern University College of Pharmacy in Ada. They may be too drying and irritating to your already parched skin. Stick with mild soaps and don't scrub too hard when you wash.

Follow the rules. While the memory of your burn is still painfully fresh, brush up on your sun sense with these tips from experts.

Apply a sunscreen about 30 minutes before going out, even if it's overcast. (Harmful rays can penetrate cloud cover.) Don't forget to protect your lips, hands, ears and the back of your neck. Reapply as necessary after swimming or perspiring heavily. Be sure to take extra care between the hours of 10:00 A.M. and 3:00 P.M. (11:00 A.M. and 4:00 P.M., daylight saving time), when the sun is at its hottest.

If you insist upon getting a tan, do so very gradually. Start with 15 minutes' exposure and increase it only a few minutes at a time. And always wear protective clothing when not swimming or sunbathing. Hats, tightly woven fabrics and long sleeves help keep the sun off your skin.

TEMPOROMANDIBULAR JOINT DISORDER (TMD)

Temporomandibular joint disorder *is quite a mouthful—hence, doctors and patients alike refer to it as TMD. But if you've got it, *pronouncing* TMD is about the easiest thing your jaws can manage.

TMD (formerly known as TMJ) is best known for its intense and debilitating pain in the temporomandibular, or jaw, joint, located in front of your ears (where sideburns are). But other ailments fall under the rubric as well: "TMD is actually a broad description for a lot of different problems in the entire facial area," says Wilmington, Delaware, dentist Barry Kayne, D.D.S., clinical assistant professor at the University of Pennsylvania School of Dental Medicine and Temple University School of Dentistry, both in Philadelphia, and a TMD specialist. "More frequent symptoms include pain in the temple, in the cheeks, behind the eyes, in the back teeth or in the throat. There may also be a popping or clicking of the jaws, neck stiffness, stuffiness in the nasal passages, ringing in the ears and migrainelike headaches . . . really bad pain throughout the entire face."

Whether brought on by growth problems, arthritis or trauma (whiplash, a sock in the jaw or other types of stretching and pummeling), TMD is common: As many as one in three people has it in some form. Sometimes TMD causes occasional jaw pain. For other people, it may be the root cause of earaches or unexplained headaches. Many people with full-fledged TMD suffer from headache—the kind of headache that creates a terrible pain in the sideburn area. If you suspect that you have TMD, here's how you may ease your discomfort.

Give your jaw R and R. "The best home remedy for TMD is to manage your jaw as you would manage a bad knee that's been injured: Provide as much rest for the area as possible, and avoid aggravating the area," says Dr. Kayne. That means you should avoid *all* unnecessary jaw movements when you're talking or eating. And you should avoid the extensive jaw movements that go along with singing or even yawning.

Stop that yawn. If you feel a yawn coming, restrict it by placing your fist under your chin, advises TMD specialist Andrew S. Kaplan, D.M.D., associate clinical professor of dentistry at Mount Sinai School of Medicine in New York City.

Unclench your teeth. If you clench your teeth, as do many people who have TMD, practice this tactic: Place your tongue behind your top front teeth so that it rests against the roof of your mouth, suggests Owen J. Rogal, D.D.S., director of the Pain Center, a multidisciplinary medical center in Philadelphia, and past executive director of the American Academy of Head, Facial and Neck Pain. This position helps separate your top and bottom teeth and relaxes your jaw.

Here's why it helps: Many people react to stressful situations by clenching their teeth, according to Dr. Kayne. "Although stress doesn't cause TMD, it certainly aggravates it," he says. "Making a conscious effort to keep your lips together and your teeth apart in stressful situations certainly helps if you have TMD."

Check your body position. If you work at a desk, check your body position throughout the day. Make sure you—and especially your chin—are not leaning over the desk, advises Dr. Rogal. As a general guideline for sitting or standing, your cheekbone should be over your clavicle, and your ears should not be too far in front of your shoulders, he says.

Many people with TMD also have back problems. The two are interrelated, Dr. Rogal says, not two separate problems.

Position a pillow . . . so you sleep on your back. Sleeping on your side or stomach puts pressure on one side of your jaw—and that causes TMD pain, says Dr. Kayne. He recommends a special cervical pillow that will help keep you on your back. "A doctor or physical therapist can tell you the best thickness for you; for most people, it's medium," says Dr. Kayne.

Get heated up. When your jaw, head or neck feels achy, apply a heating pad to ease pain. The heat increases blood flow and helps break up muscle pain, according to Dr. Kayne.

Or cool down. When the pain comes along in hard spasms, icing the area is the prescribed therapy, says Dr. Kayne. "Put an ice bag on for ten minutes, then remove it for ten minutes—and continue this process for an hour," he says. *Note:* A bag of frozen vegetables works just as well.

Take a pain reliever. Aspirin is a "marvelous" drug for any muscle or joint problem—including TMD, says Harold T. Perry, D.D.S., Ph.D., past president of the American Academy of Craniomandibular Disorders and professor of orthodontics at Northwestern University Dental School in Chicago. Ibuprofen is also recommended. "If you go that route, take aspirin or ibuprofen three or four times a day for 10 to 20 days," says Dr. Kayne. "But be consistent. Once you start, don't interrupt taking the pain reliever unless you notice stomach irritation. And also take a pain reliever *after* a meal." (And remember not to give aspirin to children because of the risk of Reye's syndrome.)

Eat soft. Whenever TMD acts up, your diet should calm down. "Don't eat anything chewy, crunchy or hard for 6 to 12 weeks," says Dr. Kayne. "That means *everything* you eat should be cooked or baked. Eat only *very* ripe fruits and vegetables. No gum, nuts, pizza, bagels, rolls, steaks—nothing that works your jaw." After ten days on a soft diet, you should notice some relief. However, Dr. Kayne advises continuing for a full 12 weeks. "If your condition doesn't improve substantially after that, see your doctor," he says.

THINNING HAIR

Father Time should get most of the blame for thinning hair. The average person loses about 100 strands per day (while the average hair grows only ½ inch per month). So the more days you live, the more hairs you lose.

But heredity is also a factor. In some families, there's a pattern of male baldness. (To a lesser degree, women in the same family can also have thinning hair.)

While you can't stop time or heredity, you can do something about the way your hair appears, even if it's thinning. Here's how.

Alter your hair hue. "Coloring your hair makes it look thicker, because as part of the coloring process, you actually 'rough up' the hair," says John Corbett, Ph.D., vice president of technology for Clairol, based in Stamford, Connecticut. He explains that it's easier to retain the appearance of fullness "because hairs don't slide over one another and lie flat against one another."

If you have extremely thin hair, go for a lighter color. "Dark colors show more of a contrast between hair and your scalp, whereas lighter colors—particularly shades of blond—hide the scalp more easily," says Dr. Corbett.

Go for the curly look. Getting a permanent wave also makes hair appear thicker, because the surface is altered (as it is in coloring) and the "wave" in the perm makes hair appear fuller.

Blow it dry. "Using a blow dryer can make hair look two to three times thicker than styling it with water or styling oils—and it *doesn't* harm the scalp, as some people believe," says Douglas D. Altchek, M.D., assistant clinical professor of dermatology at Mount Sinai School of Medicine in New York City. "When you blow-dry your hair, you plump it up, so it looks higher." Like hair coloring, blow-drying also roughs up hair shafts, so they appear thicker and fuller. But hold the dryer more than three inches away from your hair to prevent excessive dryness. Also use conditioner after your shampoo when you regularly blow-dry your hair.

BALD IS BEAUTIFUL

Some men worry that thinning hair represents lost youth and vitality. But there are a few guys—some 25,000, at least—who firmly believe that less is quite a bit more.

"The good Lord created only a few perfect heads, and the rest he covered with hair," says John T. Capps III, founder of Bald-Headed Men of America (BHMA), an international group that dedicates itself to helping the hairless.

BHMA got its start in 1972 when John lost a sales job because, the boss said, he looked too old. "I figured if it happened to me, it possibly happened to a lot of others." So John began asking his bald friends if they'd like to band together for mutual support. They said yes, and today BHMA has members in 50 states and 39 foreign countries.

Not surprisingly, the group is headquartered at 102 Bald Drive in Morehead City, North Carolina. Members attend an annual convention where they participate in self-help sessions and regale themselves with bald jokes. On a more serious note, they visit hospitals and pass out "Bald Is Beautiful" buttons, T-shirts and balloons to children who have lost their hair during cancer treatments.

John acknowledges that there are a lot of men who are embarrassed to be bald. "There's a billion-dollar industry out there, and it plays on the vanity of those individuals." But the men in BHMA, he says, "don't believe in drugs, plugs or rugs."

Wash it daily with protein shampoo. When hair is oily, it gets stringy looking. "Washing hair every day gets the oils out of it. Daily shampooing also gives hair more body, so it looks thicker right off the bat," says Harry Roth, M.D., clinical professor of dermatology at the University of California, San Francisco. "When you wash your hair with shampoo containing hydrolyzed animal proteins—also called thickeners—it actually gives hair *more diameter*."

Adds Dr. Altchek: "These hydrolyzed animal proteins coat hair so that each hair shaft is two to three times as full as it usually is. They also make hair more fluffy, which makes it appear fuller."

Use a "kitchen" conditioner. One of the best conditioners for those with thin hair is white vinegar—that's right, the same kind you use in cooking. Mix one tablespoon of white kitchen vinegar in a pint of water and massage it into your hair after shampooing, says Dr. Roth. "It changes the chemical balance of your hair to be slightly more acidic; for some reason, that makes hair appear thicker and gives it more shine. The vinegar *doesn't* leave an odor in your hair," he adds. (But of course, be sure to rinse it out before you step from the shower.)

Be an egghead. Another kitchen item that can contribute to thicker hair is the lowly egg. Simply crack an egg over your hair before shampooing, and toss away the shell. "Massage it in for five minutes and then rinse it out," adds Dr. Roth. Since egg is basically animal protein (albeit *non*hydrolyzed), it has the same effect as the specially formulated shampoos.

Go light on commercial brand conditioners. Commercial conditioners do a good job of making hair look fuller, as long as you don't overuse them. "Most people use way too much conditioner, which makes hair limp and more likely to nap together—and that makes it look even *thinner*," says Dr. Altchek. Don't use more than a teaspoonful each time you wash—that's just a dab in the palm of your hand.

Manage with mousse. A daily application of styling mousse is another way to make hair look fuller. "Since mousses have resins, they coat the hair and add diameter to it," says Dr. Corbett. Mousse lifts the hair off the scalp, which also adds to the appearance of fullness.

TOOTH STAINS

About the only thing that shines on game shows more than those fabulous showcase prizes are the smiles of the hosts. But while Wink and Chip and Skip and the rest of those hosts have a staff of makeup artists to make sure their smiles are whiter than the Arctic landscape, the rest of us regular folks have only ourselves to keep our teeth stain-free.

And sometimes, that can be harder than Double Jeopardy. Some stains can be handled only by a professional—specifically those caused by the use of certain antibiotics, a high fever or quirks in metabolism. But if you just have day-to-day problems with stained-looking teeth, there are everyday things you can do to improve them.

"Stained teeth are caused by a lot of the things we like: coffee, tea, colas, smoking, even the foods we eat. The obvious suggestion is to give up those things, but that's easier said than done for most people," explains Barry Dale, D.M.D., an Englewood, New Jersey, cosmetic dentist and assistant clinical professor at Mount Sinai Medical Center in New York City. "Even things we *don't* do can lead to staining. Teeth get more yellow as part of the natural aging process."

But some of the staining can be avoided or removed if you follow this advice.

Make water your chaser. Since coffee, tea and cola—some of our most consumed beverages—cause most of the staining in our diets, caffeine consumers can offset some of the discoloration by swishing water *after* each cup or glass. "Ideally, you can prevent many stains from forming by brushing after each meal or snack," says David S. Halpern, D.M.D., a dentist in Columbia, Maryland, and a spokesperson for the Academy of General Dentistry. "But since most people don't do that, I advise my patients to take a cup of water and swish it around after they drink coffee or another staining beverage. Besides diminishing the initial film stain of coffee, it also helps keep their breath relatively fresh."

"BLEACHING" KITS CLEAN WALLETS MORE THAN TEETH

Thinking about using one of those tooth polishes advertised on TV that promise you a mouthful of pearly whites? If you go ahead and spend your money for those products, you're being shucked like an oyster.

"Some are so abrasive that while they may initially appear to whiten your teeth, they can make them even darker, because they strip away the enamel—leaving the darker dentin exposed," says Barry Dale, D.M.D., an Englewood, New Jersey, cosmetic dentist and assistant clinical professor at Mount Sinai Medical Center in New York City. "What happens is that you turn your slightly yellowed teeth a darker color."

And dark teeth are only the beginning of your problems if you begin using these polishing gels, pastes and other "bleaching" kits. New evidence suggests that they can be harmful to your health. "Some studies suggest they may potentiate other cancer-causing agents," says Dr. Dale. "That means if you smoke, for instance, using bleaching kits may enhance the risk of mouth cancer."

Eat a lot of crunchy foods. "Consuming apples, celery and other crunchy foods that rub against the teeth helps dislodge debris that can cause staining," adds Dr. Halpern. "I notice more of a staining problem in patients who eat a lot of sticky foods."

Keep peroxide for cleaning wounds, not teeth. True, dentists use a peroxide solution to bleach stained teeth. But that doesn't mean you can do it yourself with store-bought varieties. "What we use is a special 35 percent peroxide solution that's very strong," says Dr. Dale. "There's no evidence that rinsing with the 2 percent peroxide you buy at the drugstore will help keep teeth white."

Don't brush too hard. Logic might suggest that the harder you brush, the cleaner you'll get your teeth. But reality says otherwise. "Brushing too vigorously can actually strip some of the enamel off teeth, exposing the darker inner layer called the dentin," says Dr. Dale. His advice: Brush your teeth firmly but not vigorously—and use only soft-bristle brushes, not those with medium or hard bristles. "If you can't remove the stain with regular brushing and toothpaste, then you won't remove it by brushing harder."

Check your plaque quotient. Rinse with a disclosing solution to show where plaque remains on your teeth after brushing. Those spots are where your teeth will stain if you don't improve your brushing technique, says John D.B. Featherstone, Ph.D., chairman of the Department of Oral Biology at the Eastman Dental Center in Rochester, New York.

Electrify your smile. An electric toothbrush, says Ronald I. Maitland, D.M.D., who specializes in cosmetic dentistry in his New York City practice, will push more of the stain-collecting plaque off your teeth. Studies show an electric toothbrush can remove 98.2 percent of plaque.

INDEX

Note: <u>Underscored</u> page references indicate boxed text.